COPING
WITH A
*H*YSTERECTOMY

COPING
WITH A
HYSTERECTOMY

your own choice, your own solutions

Susanne Morgan

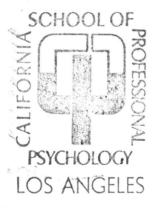

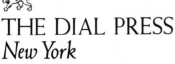

THE DIAL PRESS
New York

Published by
The Dial Press
1 Dag Hammarskjold Plaza
New York, New York 10017

Manufactured in the United States of America

First printing

Library of Congress Cataloging in Publication Data

Morgan, Susanne.
   Coping with a hysterectomy.

   Includes bibliographies and index.
   1. Hysterectomy.   2. Hysterectomy—Psychological
aspects.   I. Title.
RG391.M67   618.1'453   81-15122
ISBN 0-385-27215-4   AACR2

To David and Catherine

CONTENTS

FOREWORD

Choice is the voluntary action of picking, singling out, or select-
ing from two or more that which is favored or superior. It is the
freedom to decide.

Hysterectomy is the most common major operation performed
in the U.S. It has been projected that within the next several
years, gynecologic surgeons will have removed the uteruses of
one-half of the women in the U.S., so many more than that number will at least be faced with the possibility of having a
hysterectomy.

Does a woman have a choice about hysterectomy? What information is available to her? What are the fears as well as the
medical and psychological conditions of the woman who must
choose? How many women are told by their doctors, "I have no
choice. I must remove your uterus." How many women know
if or why their ovaries are also going to be removed during
surgery?

To choose that which is superior implies knowledge of the

options and consequences. That knowledge has been primarily in the hands of the medical profession and only reluctantly made accessible to women.

I have often thought that in every doctor's office, a nurse should ask the patient who has just been seen, "Do you understand what has just occurred in this office? Do you know what is wrong? Do you know what treatments are recommended or planned?" and finally, "Do you have any questions?" However, it has never been the intent of the medical profession to empower women with knowledge about their bodies or choices in what procedures are performed upon them.

A physician writes about the six types of "pesky patients" who drive him "up the wall," including the "insolvent inquirer." She is a woman having her first baby, "and she intends to approach it the way Einstein approached relativity." Then he tells us, "She didn't get straight [A's] at Vassar for nothing." This woman's crime was to have questions about natural childbirth, analgesia, anesthesia, methods of delivery, and finally cost.*

Thirty percent of women between the ages of thirty-five and seventy-four have already had a hysterectomy. That high prevalence rate in itself makes it more difficult for a woman to say no, or even to consider saying no. If a woman's mother, sisters, aunts, friends, have had hysterectomies, then it becomes more difficult for any one woman to say, "But I do not want to have my uterus removed." The surgery gains legitimacy by being so commonly performed. Hysterectomy is as much a part of an adult woman's life as tonsillectomy is for a child's. Losing one's uterus becomes a cultural expectation.

It is also difficult for a woman to feel a sense of choice about hysterectomy because often she is faced with a decision at a time she is not feeling well. Illness and fear are not conducive to free choice. Frightened, bleeding, fearful of cancer, women are not in a good position to demand answers to questions or sometimes even to ask them. There is a natural tendency when sick

---

* Kenneth R. Morgan. "Must You Coax Her in Lithotomy Position?" *Medical Economics* (Dec. 13, 1976):201–204.

to want to trust the judgment of others, to let oneself be taken care of. It is even more difficult for the woman who is already in the hospital when she is told she needs a hysterectomy. Lying in a hospital bed, separated from clothes, support, and the props which represent one's own sense of strength, it is difficult to challenge what the experts standing around are saying. Hospitals are infantilizing.

Susanne Morgan gives women more of a choice. By presenting a vast amount of information about hysterectomy, both medical beliefs and the experiences of women who have had the surgery, she enables the reader to understand what the operation is, when and why it is performed, and what are its consequences. In the words of women, she presents the real sequelae and reactions to hysterectomy.

"How will I feel?" cannot be answered by the doctor advising removal of a woman's uterus—and possibly her ovaries too—but many women answer that question in this book. For the first time, in a way similar to *The Hite Report*, women describe what it was like, not what they think they should have experienced.

Although 100 years ago women underwent hysterectomy and ovariectomy for excess sexual urges, today women are told that such surgery will have no effect on their sexual experiences. But the women to whom Susanne Morgan spoke and listened refute that notion. There are changes, some good, some bad, some just different, but changes there are!

Susanne Morgan says that if you are told you need a hysterectomy, you should be certain you really need it, since there are many unnecessary ones performed. Then, she says, if you must have it, this is what it will be like, before the surgery, during recovery, and in the months and years that follow. Free of judgment as to whether any woman should have or should not have had her hysterectomy, she calls for an understanding that every decision can only be made with the best information at hand at the time. No woman should punish herself for a decision which becomes questionable in retrospect.

Susanne Morgan also makes real the choice about hysterectomy by presenting some alternatives. She discusses ways in which women can improve their general health and capacity for self-healing to counteract some of the less desirable effects of hysterectomy and ovariectomy.

This book is for everyone. It is to be read by every woman who has had or may still have a hysterectomy, as well as for any man who would like to be more sensitive and supportive of women whose lives are touched by hysterectomy.

Throughout the book, Susanne Morgan admonishes women to speak to each other, to break the silence that has left each woman wondering why she feels as she does, why she isn't reacting as she was told she should. In this book, the facts are presented, experiences are shared, and a conspiracy of silence is broken. Women's voices prevail.

—MICHELLE HARRISON, M.D.,

PREFACE

This book is the result of the convergence of three parts of my life. Professionally, I am a medical sociologist. I teach and consult primarily in the area of health policy. My Ph.D. from Case Western Reserve University was awarded in 1972, and I have been teaching in universities, in Boston and California, since that time. I like the way medical sociology and sociology about women's health help us understand both interpersonal relationships and our personal feelings as well as social trends and the implications of policies. The most exciting teaching I have done has been courses on women's health policy.

Politically, I have become very active in women's health issues outside the university. I am a founding member of the California Women's Health Network, and have been active in the National Women's Health Network. I try to keep up-to-date on what is happening in a wide variety of struggles for human rights in the health area. At an interpersonal level I teach re-evaluation co-counseling, which is a way of energizing individuals for more effective functioning in society. I am concerned about social problems and try to help bring about social change.

My interest in hysterectomy, though, came about because of personal experience. In 1974 I developed a pelvic infection from an IUD (intrauterine device) that had been inserted after my second child was born. Despite many courses of antibiotics, the infection never cleared up. I was sick for twelve months with pain and a fever, and had several operations during that time. In the end I had a hysterectomy and ovariectomy. The surgery was in 1975, when I was thirty years old. Within the options and information available to me then, the hysterectomy was necessary. I had an excellent recovery, and my general state of health has continued to improve since that time.

At that time very little had been written about hysterectomy, and even less from the perspective I think is important. I began to read about it in the literature of research medicine, clinical medicine, psychology, nursing, and epidemiology. I presented talks and support groups on hysterectomy and menopause, acted as a counselor and advocate for women going through a hysterectomy decision.

I have written several articles: one on sexuality for the journal *Women and Health,* one for the journal *HealthRight,* called "War on the Womb," and a twenty-page pamphlet that was published by The Boston Women's Health Book Collective, the authors of the book *Our Bodies, Ourselves.* The pamphlet is now included as part of the hysterectomy resource guide available from the National Women's Health Network. This book is an expansion of those projects, to make their material more widely available to more women.

If you are considering a hysterectomy, you want to know more about the condition doctors say you have, and what the various options may be, as well as the real risks and hazards you may encounter. You need questions to ask the doctor, to help you get and clarify the information you need. The ways other women have handled the decision and feelings they have had while making it will also be helpful. The words of women who have come through the surgery and are now active, strong, and happy can be reassuring. It can be comforting to know that other women have had the fears and feelings you are experiencing and that you are not "neurotic" for having them. If you want to hold out and avoid a hysterectomy, the specific ways that other women have avoided surgery can provide inspiration.

If you have already had a hysterectomy, you may want to know whether your experiences are like those of other women and whether they could be related to your surgery. Sometimes it can be a relief to be given permission to express many different feelings, such as rage and grief and glee, about your surgery. Whether you are among the women for whom the surgery was easy, wonderful, the best thing that ever happened to you, or among those who feel bitter and angry about it, all of those experiences are true and real and you can be proud of them. If your ovaries have been removed, you need information about estrogen. Should you take it? What are the dangers? What have other women done about the decision? You want to know ways to be a more alert health care consumer.

You may be involved with women having hysterectomies through one of the helping professions, such as nursing, counseling, clergy, or medicine. A friend or family member may be considering or have had a hysterectomy. If you understand the many varieties of experiences women have, you will be better able to support the woman you care about. You may also want more information to share with the person you care about, to help her find more answers on her own.

Hysterectomy is also a policy issue. It is important to people working on lawsuits or regulations regarding surgery. Activists for women's rights or the rights of minorities, and students choosing the topic of hysterectomy because it has personal and social significance are concerned as well.

Three themes underlie my analysis of hysterectomy. First, we need more information, as health care consumers, if we are working in the health care profession, or if we are researchers. Second, we should talk with one another. Other women are invaluable sources of information and support. Third, whatever the outcome of your personal experience, you always do the very best you can in your situation. Even if you later regret the decision you made, you made the very best decision you could in the circumstances you found yourself in. You will find I am extremely critical of the very high rate of hysterectomy, and yet very supportive of every woman I know who has had a hysterectomy.

In the book I include notes to technical sources at the end. Because so much medical information is presented to us in a watered-down version, I want my sources to be accessible to you.

As I write, women's voices echo in my mind. Voices of support and encouragement, and voices telling their stories. Some of the voices and some of the stories are included in the book, and you will each have your own to add. I have changed names and sometimes situations for confidentiality.

ACKNOWLEDGMENTS

Countless people have played a part in this project. Women who attended workshops, who shared their experiences with me, and who insisted the book must be written, all remain in my mind. My friends and support network, who kept me working and healing, continue to sustain me. Patricia Potter has, over the years, typed the entire manuscript at least twice and cheered me on. Specifically, the following people read chapters: Norma Swenson, M.P.H. ("Rates and Risks"; "War on the Womb"), Marjorie Buck, R.N. ("What's a Woman to Do?"; "Taking It Out"), Karen Anderson, Ph.D. ("Feelings, Fears, and Grief"), Edith Bjornson Sunley ("Sexuality"), and Barbara Seaman ("Home-Brew Estrogen"). Finally, Khandiz Ayofemi Stowe read the entire manuscript and provided unfailing support and nurture.

COPING
WITH A
HYSTERECTOMY

Chapter One

WHAT IS HYSTERECTOMY?

What is hysterectomy? The mixed and emotionally charged messages most of us have received when the word is mentioned have often prevented real information from coming through. The atmosphere of hush and secret has kept us from thinking clearly about it.

In addition to the emotional barrier to communication, very little solid information has been made available to most of us. Most women say their doctors have not explained as fully as they would like what their health situation is or what the surgery would mean. Women who have received sufficient information feel very fortunate that they have an exceptional doctor. Doctors are not trained for patient-education. Their training is in diagnosis and treatment or in surgery, and communicating information clearly is not their strong point. Frequently they assume that too much information will confuse or disturb a woman, or that she will be unable to understand it. This obviously reinforces women's feelings of inadequacy concerning the question of hysterectomy.

When I ask women what they think hysterectomy means, I get a variety of answers:

"You can't have babies."
"Your womb is taken out."
"Your ovaries, they clean you out."
"I think a partial is better than a total."
"No, a partial leaves things in and you might have to have another operation."

Briefly, hysterectomy is the removal of a woman's uterus. Generally her cervix is removed as well. If her ovaries are removed, it is called ovariectomy or oophorectomy. The second term is pronounced "o' a fer ec' to me," or "oo' fer ec' to me." If the ovaries are removed, the fallopian tubes are usually removed also. We often refer to this procedure as "total hysterectomy," but the technical term is "panhysterectomy with bilateral salpingo-oophorectomy." "Pan" means the uterus and cervix, "salpinges" or "salpinx" are the tubes, and "bilateral" means both sides. The suffix "ectomy" means removal.

"Partial" hysterectomy sometimes means removing only the uterus and not the ovaries; sometimes it means the uterus and not the cervix. Since women and health professionals use a variety of meanings for it, I generally do not use the term "partial."

The diagrams on pages 5 and 6 show a woman's pelvic structure. Our uterus, or womb, is the organ in which a baby can grow and where our menstrual flow originates. Our vagina is the channel that leads from the uterus to the outside of the body. The cervix is the portion of the uterus that extends into the vagina. It has a small opening called the os, which opens wide during childbirth. The menstrual flow comes through the os.

The ovaries produce hormones that go into the bloodstream. They also produce an egg more or less monthly (ovulation) between puberty and menopause, except when we are pregnant

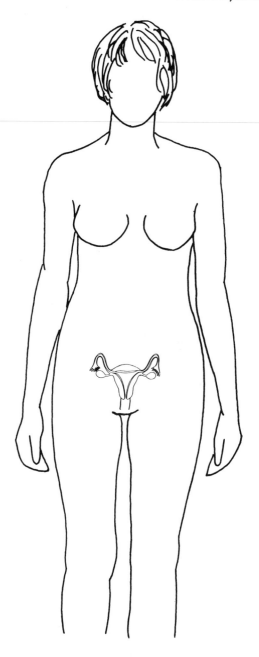

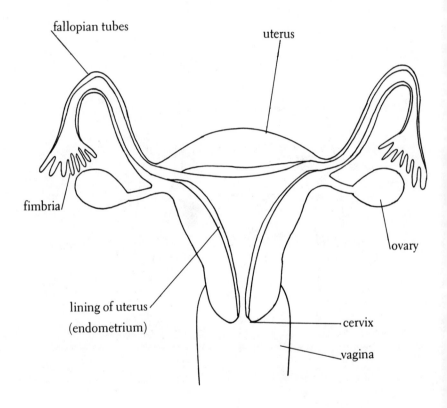

fallopian tubes

uterus

fimbria

ovary

lining of uterus
(endometrium)

cervix

vagina

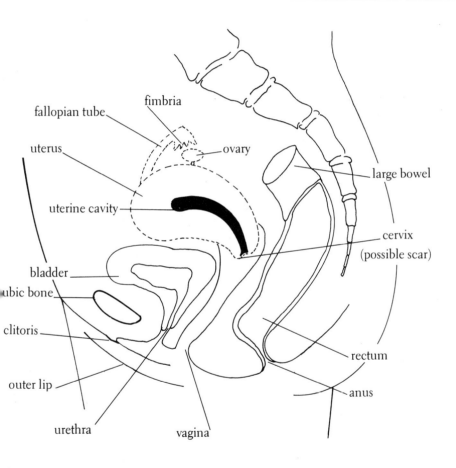

Female pelvic organs.
Organs removed in hysterectomy are indicated with dotted lines.

or nursing or taking birth control pills. The fallopian tubes carry the egg to the uterus. Menstruation follows unless sperm fertilizes the egg, making us pregnant.

After hysterectomy, we will not have menstrual periods and we will not become pregnant. We will, however, still have our monthly hormone cycles, unless our ovaries are removed. We will have our vagina and can still have sex. Page 7 shows the pelvis after hysterectomy. If our ovaries are removed, our hormone level changes very suddenly and we experience "instant menopause," which I call "menostop," unless we have gone through menopause already.

As you look at the diagram, note some things you may not have known before. One is that the ovaries are not attached to the fallopian tubes. They "float" in the pelvic cavity. Also notice that the cervix is actually part of the uterus. It extends into the vagina and feels like the tip of a nose if you reach your finger up into your vagina.

After the uterus is removed the other organs of the pelvic cavity move around to fill in the space it occupied.

WHAT IS CASTRATION?

I have never talked with a woman who was told she would be castrated, and yet many of us were. Perhaps you were. Ask people what they think castration means, and you will get a variety of responses. You will also get many blank stares and suddenly pale faces:

"It's when they take a man's penis off?"
"No, it's when they take his testicles."

"Can they castrate a woman?"
"Is hysterectomy castration?"
"Is castration if they take away the vagina?"
"Is it when her ovaries are removed?"

Castration means removing a woman's ovaries. It is parallel to removing a man's testicles. Another term for removing the ovaries is surgical menopause. After her ovaries are removed, a woman will be in a state very much like menopause. I call it menostop because it happens so very suddenly.

The feelings aroused by the term "castration" are very strong, and that makes it hard to think clearly. After castration an adult man can perform sexually, but he requires more time to reach an erection. The same is true with a woman. Some of us think hysterectomy always includes removing the ovaries. Others think if the ovaries are removed we become eunuchs and have no sex life. Neither of those ideas is true. Hysterectomy itself includes only removing the uterus. If the ovaries are removed, it is either because they too are diseased or because they should be removed for some other reason. Some diseases involve hormone production, so part of the treatment would include removing the ovaries. This is true for severe and advanced endometriosis (see page 17) or breast cancer in some cases.

If a woman is clearly past the menopause already, the consensus is that the ovaries probably should be removed; if she is younger, the choice is less clear. Even this medical opinion may change as more research suggests that the ovaries do have a function after menopause.

Doctors sometimes suggest removing the ovaries to prevent ovarian cancer. Although ovarian cancer grows quickly and is hard to detect, it still represents only 1 percent of all cancers. Only 4 to 10 percent of women with ovarian cancer had previously had a hysterectomy, so only for those women would removing the ovaries have prevented cancer. Follow-up studies of hysterectomy patients show that very few actually develop ovarian cancer.

If a premenopausal woman must have an ovariectomy because of illness, menostop has a major effect. The levels of estrogen and progesterone, the hormones produced by the ovaries, drop very suddenly. As our bodies adjust to the new level, we will probably have very severe hot flashes—brief periods of extreme heat and sometimes perspiration. We may also have headaches, irritability, or fatigue. As our bodies adjust to the loss of the ovaries, some changes may remain. We may have changes in body hair, less pubic hair or more facial hair. We may find a change in skin texture, and our labia (the fleshy lips of the vulva or genital area) may shrink somewhat.

We may also notice changes in our sexual experiences. The walls of the vagina may become thinner, we may have less vaginal lubrication, and it may take longer to become lubricated.

Some researchers think menopause may be related to osteoporosis, a condition in which the bones become brittle and break easily and the back can become fused in a "dowager's hump," but this relationship is unclear. Part of the controversy about whether to take estrogen replacement therapy revolves around whether osteoporosis is prevented by taking estrogens.

One bit of good news about ovariectomy is that women who experience premature menopause have a very low rate of breast cancer.

For those of us who are physically postmenopausal before we are socially defined as middle-aged, the experience is also different. Women who go through surgical menopause are more likely to identify changes they notice as being results of the surgical menopause rather than as being personal changes related to aging. I wonder if those women who are castrated in their twenties or thirties may have a somewhat easier time in their forties and fifties, since the physical changes will have occurred already.

However, because menostop is so sudden and so early, women have far more drastic changes to cope with. Furthermore, we do not know whether being postmenopausal for forty to fifty years rather than twenty to thirty years may bring about unexpected problems.

Hysterectomy and castration are important topics for women

today. If, as some researchers predict, one-half of all women in the United States will eventually have a hysterectomy, many more of us will be offered a hysterectomy and will decline. So the topic will be relevant for a majority of women in this country and for those who care about those women.

Chapter Two

PROBLEMS and ALTERNATIVES

The major indications (the medical term for reasons) for hysterectomy range from life-threatening illness to sterilization or prevention of disease. In fact very few hysterectomies are done in response to life-threatening problems. Even the 8 to 12 percent of hysterectomies that are performed to treat gynecological cancers may not all be necessary. With respect to the other causes, there is a great deal of controversy and uncertainty about when hysterectomies are truly necessary.

FIBROIDS

Fibroids may be the most common reason for hysterectomy, as they account for 27 to 33 percent of the total number performed. "Fibroids" is the common term for benign tumors that are medically known as myomas or leiomyomas. They grow in the muscle tissue of the uterus.

Fibroids are very common. One woman in four or five develops them, and for some reason black women seem to get fibroids more often than white women. Having a fibroid does not mean you need a hysterectomy. You may have fibroids and never know it at all. Small fibroids can cause some symptoms, such as a feeling of heaviness in the pelvic area, or irregular or heavy menstrual bleeding, or pain in the bladder or rectum. If you go back to the drawing of the pelvic cavity, you will see that the uterus lies very close to the bladder and the rectum. It will be closer to one or the other depending on which way it is tipped or lying in the pelvic cavity. If it is enlarged because of fibroids, it can press on the bladder or rectum, causing discomfort or pain.

Fibroids generally grow very slowly. They are also related to estrogen, and they shrink in size during menopause. If you have fibroids that are beginning to give you trouble but you are forty-eight years old, you might be able to last it out until menopause shrinks the fibroids. If you are twenty-eight and the fibroids are giving you a great deal of trouble, then your costs and benefits will appear in a different light.

Because fibroids are affected by estrogen, if you are taking estrogen replacement drugs or have recently been taking birth control pills and discover the fibroids are growing more rapidly, it might make sense to stop the estrogen and see what happens. If fibroids grow rapidly without estrogen drugs, they would arouse medical concern about the possibility of a precancerous condition.

You may be told that you have a subserous fibroid, or an intramural fibroid or a submucosal fibroid. This simply refers to where in the uterus the fibroid is growing. Subserous fibroids grow in the lining between the uterus and the outside pelvic cavity, intramural fibroids lie within the walls of the uterus, and submucosal fibroids grow into the uterine cavity from the endometrium, or the lining of the uterus.

How do you decide if your fibroids are giving you sufficient trouble that a hysterectomy would make sense? Because fibroids are always benign, and because they are so very common, clear answers are difficult. The statisticians generally use a decision based on the size of the fibroids: in one study a leiomyoma with a uterine weight of over 200 grams represented a justifiable hysterectomy. Doctors in practice sometimes judge the size of a fibroid by comparing the size of the uterus with the size of a pregnant uterus. One doctor, for example, judges a fibroid to be too large if it makes the uterus larger than it would be at sixteen weeks of pregnancy.

For any individual woman the first consideration will be whether she has any difficulties. Doctors can use existing fibroids as a reason to talk a woman into a hysterectomy. One basic scare tactic is the use of the word "tumor." Fibroids are indeed tumors, and we usually think "cancer" when we hear the word "tumor." Fibroids, however, are not cancer and do not threaten our lives. Yet the term is often consciously used to elicit the fear of cancer and prompt the woman to agree to hysterectomy.

When asked by a researcher what he would do with nine to ten week sized asymptomatic fibroids, a fourth-year resident answered:

> Uh, most likely I would do the surgery. . . . I would explain to her that she has fibroids that are nine to ten weeks sized, that she isn't going to have a family anymore, she doesn't want a family anymore, that these fibroids *may* sometime in the future grow bigger, *may* get symptoms, *may* cause

her trouble, she *may* need surgery at some point in time, and if she would like to have surgery done now it can be easy surgery, vaginally. As a consequence, she won't have any more children, but she won't have any fibroids and she won't have any potential for disease. [Researcher: Put like that, many people would say yes.] Right, but is that being dishonest? [Researcher: Those fibroids may also disappear by themselves.] Right, but you are only saying they may do this or they may do that and essentially you let the patient make up her mind. Usually when patients hear they have fibroids and there is some bleeding, there is a sufficient symptomatology.

If you are not aware of difficulties from your fibroids, you almost certainly do not need to think in terms of surgery. If you have difficulties, you have plenty of time to embark on some alternative healing efforts or at least seek an additional medical opinion.

A medical alternative for fibroids can be an operation called myomectomy. Myomectomy is surgical removal of the fibroid tumor itself. Sometimes this is not possible, particularly if the fibroid has grown within the walls of the uterus. Hysterectomy is a more commonly performed and easier operation for doctors to do. It is hard to find doctors who are familiar and practiced at doing myomectomy.

Doctors are taught to suggest myomectomy only if the woman has not had the children she wants. This is one of the ways in which doctors' judgment about women's roles may interfere with good medical practice. It may be that for many women myomectomy makes the most sense. Yet doctors' assumptions are that the uterus has only one function and that is reproduction. Although certainly it is important to retain our childbearing capacity if we want to have children, medical practice should not be based on the assumption that the uterus is useless except for childbearing and that it has no symbolic significance and no physical sensation. In fact, the uterus has many functions, including sexual ones.

Infertility experts estimate the success rate of myomectomy for future pregnancies at 30 to 60 percent. A myomectomy may not insure future pregnancies, but it will preserve the uterus and its other functions.

If you have fibroids that are giving you trouble and you want to investigate myomectomy, look for a specialist on infertility. Even if you have had all the children you want or have no difficulties with fertility, infertility specialists may be more aware of alternatives to hysterectomy for fibroids.

A recently introduced surgical treatment for fibroids involves "shaving" them off with an instrument called a hysterscope. This technique has been used by Dr. Robert Neuwirth of Columbia University.

Nonmedical alternatives for women with fibroids often involve cleansing fasts or long periods of modified fasting. One theory is that a fast or a modified fast reduces tumors by "starving them out."

If the fibroids are causing discomfort because of pressure on other organs, yoga exercises could be helpful. Some people have found that vitamin A is helpful in reducing heavy bleeding. Because fibroids are tumors, visualization work can be effective in reducing their size.

Enid had a hysterectomy for fibroids and is glad she did:

> My periods had been getting worse and worse for several years. They were so heavy that I was feeling very weak and anemic. My doctor didn't want to do the surgery but I shopped around until I found someone who did. I have felt nothing but relief ever since. I recovered quickly and feel strong and healthy now.

Enid's hysterectomy was probably technically unnecessary, and even her regular doctor hesitated to do it. She is glad she had it done, and she feels much better. Perhaps if more options had been commonly available, Enid would have chosen a different course. But hysterectomy appeared to her to be the best option of those she had, and she is glad she made that decision.

Jean tried a different route.

> My fibroids made my uterus the size of a sixteen-week fetus
> and the doctors were all talking about hysterectomy. For
> some reason I came across the book by Henry Bieler called
> *Food Is Your Best Medicine.* I put together my own diet,
> mostly steamed vegetables and a little fish. If I see another
> zucchini, I think I'll die. But my fibroids went from being
> sixteen weeks with very heavy bleeding to being eight weeks
> size and no heavy bleeding at all. At first it was very hard,
> and by the end, I was desperate to eat some other food. Now
> and then I'd slip, but in the middle part it wasn't hard at all.
> I'm already thirty-eight, so I should be going through the
> change soon. If I've got them down this far now, they
> probably won't get too big before menopause.

Marian's story is less dramatic.

> Here I am thirty-five and my fibroids are fairly large and
> I'm bleeding fairly heavily. I'm trying my best right now
> to wait and see. I've been eating better and getting more
> exercise and I'm certainly feeling better even if my fibroids
> haven't changed. They certainly are not getting worse, and
> my doctor agrees the things I'm doing for myself are prob-
> ably not going to hurt.

ENDOMETRIOSIS

The endometrium is the special tissue that lines the uterus.
It builds up each month, and then is sloughed off through the

vagina during menstruation. Of course, if an egg is fertilized, the egg is implanted in the endometrium, which does not slough off this time and is the tissue in which the fetus begins to grow during pregnancy.

Endometriosis is a disorder in which endometrial tissue grows in places other than the inside of the uterus. The portions of endometrial tissue outside the uterus are called implants. They generally are found in or on the ovaries, bladder, or rectum.

The tissue in the endometrial implants becomes engorged with blood each month, and at the time the uterine endometrial tissue is being discharged into your vagina (your menstrual period), the outside endometrial tissue bleeds into the pelvic cavity. Very little blood actually is lost, and seldom does endometriosis cause dangerous internal bleeding.

The major symptom of endometriosis is extreme menstrual pain. Many women with endometriosis also have painful ovulation, approximately halfway between menstrual periods. Some have painful intercourse. Others have no symptoms except infertility.

If you have painful menstrual periods your doctor should make sure you do not have endometriosis before proceeding with other treatments. Endometriosis is most common among younger women and women who have not had children.

Sometimes the implants grow as adhesions between two parts of the pelvic cavity, such as between an ovary and a coil of the bowel. If endometriosis causes adhesions, this produces even greater pain, because any movement by any part of the body is felt as pain in the other. For example, passing gas through the rectum could cause uterine or ovarian pain if those organs have been attached to the rectum by adhesions.

Women with endometriosis are more likely to have problems conceiving a child than women without endometriosis. For that reason, if you have endometriosis and are considering having children, you might want to evaluate whether now is the time to have children. You might want to try to find a partner, or convince your partner to have children, or decide to do it alone with artificial insemination.

If you do become pregnant, your endometriosis will probably recede. No one knows the exact cause of endometriosis, but it is known to be related to the hormone cycle. If you have not been pregnant, pregnancy will probably help your condition greatly. If you are close to menopause, menopause will also probably help the endometriosis.

If you think about the above statements, you will realize that "pseudopregnancy" or "artificial menopause" might also improve endometriosis. You are exactly right, and both of those treatments are in fact suggested for endometriosis. Hormone drugs such as birth control pills, because they prevent the release of eggs and the build-up of endometrial tissue, help to control endometriosis. A permanent cure for endometriosis is the removal of the ovaries. Between those two options is the removal of the actual implants, which sometimes can be done.

Infertility specialists recommend the following progression of treatments if a woman chooses to try to become pregnant, and these treatments probably are appropriate for any woman who prefers to avoid hysterectomy.

First, the patient is carefully observed and given pain medication for the menstrual cramping. Second, hormones are administered to suppress ovulation. After that the endometriosis may be improved sufficiently for the woman to become pregnant. Third, surgery of the implants and hormone therapy are recommended. Infertility specialists claim a 30 to 40 percent success rate in pregnancy after surgery of implants.

Hormone drugs all carry risks. Birth control pills and menopausal estrogens carry risks of blood clots, gallbladder disease, and possibly cancer. A nonestrogen drug sometimes given for endometriosis is called danazol. Danazol also has risks, called "mild" by doctors, including nausea, hot flashes, mild depression, muscle cramps, weight gain, acne, and irregular bleeding. Some androgenic (more like male) side effects, such as facial hair growth and voice changes, are reversible, but some may be permanent.

Hormone drugs, however, are less risky for most women than hysterectomy, and their effects are obviously less permanent. If you are offered hormone drugs, be sure to obtain full information about their risks. Hormones have risks of disease, including cancer, and other problems. They can also cause bleeding, which could then lead to hysterectomy. Hormones may be your true choice, but you should be very sure.

It may be possible to determine the extent of the endometriosis by laparoscopy. The instrument involved, the same one used in the "Band-Aid sterilization," is a thin tube inserted in the abdomen through a tiny incision. Gas is introduced into the abdomen to move the organs apart so they are more visible, and a light and tube to look through are inserted. Laparoscopy is an excellent next step to take if the doctor's examination has identified within the abdomen some growth whose size or exact placement is unclear. With laparoscopy it may be possible to determine the extent and nature of the implants and how much your fertility is jeopardized.

Suppose you are not interested in having children, or you know you are already infertile, and the doctor says you have endometriosis. What then? If the endometriosis is not troubling you, it is probably not necessary to do anything about it. If you do have pain, then you need to weigh your options. Perhaps the pain is so severe you are extremely debilitated for several days each month, and menopause is far away. Perhaps you have already tried drug treatments, and they have not improved your condition sufficiently. For you the risks of hysterectomy (and do be sure you have a full picture of the real risks) may be worth incurring in order to end your pain. If your pain is moderate, you may have the energy to try alternative treatments before seriously considering premature menopause and hysterectomy.

Seeking alternative treatments for a condition such as endometriosis can be a circular process. Because we are debilitated by pain and fear of significant illness, we have less energy left to seek alternative treatments. Simply going to the doctor appears to take the least energy. The catch is that the treatment suggested by the doctor is almost always more radical and perhaps more hazardous than other kinds of treatment.

Self-healing of endometriosis requires a commitment to yourself and your healing. Methods women have used include a cleansing fast monthly, with special attention to emptying the bowels fully, an exercise program including especially yoga, and visualization methods. To visualize your body as healthy and strong and beautiful, and to visualize healing energy going to your painful parts, can be powerful in endometriosis.

Ruth has endometriosis and is twenty-five. She feels very much caught in the middle with no satisfactory options.

> Nothing seems to be working. I have terrible cramps, and I want desperately to have children sometime. I'm very nervous about taking estrogen drugs, and when I have they have made me sick. Sometimes I think "Oh, well, give it up—go ahead and have a hysterectomy." But then I realize they would have me on hormone drugs for the rest of my life if I had my ovaries out, so it seems like no option is going to be very good.

Irene sent me a copy of an article from the Canadian women's health journal, *Health Sharing*. She writes:

> All I did was to get some of the books this article talks about and try some of the activities. I can tell I still have problems, but it all seems already much better. Maybe it's just because I'm feeling better, but I feel certain that I'm not going to have to have a hysterectomy.

PELVIC INFECTIONS

An increasing number of hysterectomies are performed because of severe pelvic infections. Pelvic infections are grouped together and referred to as pelvic inflammatory disease (PID). Infections can be caused by a variety of bacteria, and can attack various organs. You may be told you have endometritis (an infection of the endometrium, the lining of the uterus), parametritis (an infection of the uterus), salpingitis (an infection of the fallopian tubes), or salpingo-oophoritis (an infection of the tubes and ovaries). Recently increasing numbers of PID cases are found to be caused by the Chlamydia bacteria, and approximately 60 percent are caused by gonococcus.

The symptoms of pelvic infections are sharp or dull pelvic pain, sometimes with fever and sometimes with foul vaginal discharge. Many women find pelvic pain very easy to ignore. We are accustomed to cramps; we have been told, directly or indirectly, that pelvic pain is "in our head"; and often it is hard to put our own needs ahead of those of our family. Any pelvic pain is important. It could be an infection that if caught quickly can be fully treated, and it could be a warning of something more serious.

The rate of PID is increasing very rapidly, for two primary reasons. One is the epidemic of diseases such as gonorrhea and other sexually transmitted bacteria. Gonorrhea sometimes produces no symptoms in women until a serious infection has started. The other cause is the IUD (intrauterine device). Many studies now document the increasing incidence of infections in women using the IUD, and the risk of PID is estimated as 1.6 to 9.3 times higher in IUD wearers. One theory of the way the IUD works is that it creates a low-grade infection in the uterus, making the uterus more susceptible to bacteria. Another theory is that the bacteria may be introduced into the uterus along the string of the IUD. The tragedy of IUD-caused PID is emphasized by the fact that contraceptives like condoms and diaphragms *protect* against PID.

Because pelvic infections from IUDs are becoming so common, and because even a low-grade pelvic infection can lead to scarring of the fallopian tubes such that pregnancy is impossible, women who have not had children are being discouraged from using the IUD. Infertility as a result of the IUD is an increasing problem.

The progression of a pelvic infection, or PID, may be roughly like this: bacteria are introduced into the vagina and somehow travel into the uterus. It is likely that resistance plays a part in whether the bacteria lead to a severe infection or not. The lesson, of course, is that the healthier we are, the less likely we are to develop a major infection.

The first phase is acute PID, most common in the twenty to twenty-four age group. This will be accompanied by significant pain and probably a high fever. This stage can be very brief, however, and you could move through it without knowing it.

If PID is diagnosed at the acute stage, antibiotics are prescribed. If you take antibiotics, it is important to take them for the full length of time prescribed, even if the symptoms improve. Complete bedrest is also recommended for PID, although not everyone is told or encouraged to rest by her doctor.

If not interrupted, the next stage of PID is chronic PID. This means you have a low-grade infection with pain and probably a low or intermittent fever. At this stage the treatment is antibiotics, but it appears the chance that the infection will not respond to antibiotics is greater. Hospitalization for complete bed rest and a course of intravenously administered antibiotics in a higher dosage may be advised.

If you are taking antibiotics by mouth, be sure to take extra care of your health. Antibiotics are a great strain on the body and deplete its supply of B vitamins. Some doctors prescribe B vitamins for people taking antibiotics, and other women find that taking vitamins and eating yogurt helps while they are on antibiotics. The reason for eating yogurt is that antibiotics kill off the helpful bacteria that live in the intestines. Yogurt culture contains some of those helpful bacteria.

Laparoscopy is a useful technique with PID as well as with other pelvic problems. It can enable the doctor to see whether there are abscesses and how inflamed the tubes or ovaries or uterus appear. If your doctor recommends a hysterectomy for

PID and you have not had a laparoscopic examination, check to see whether you could have that first.

One danger with untreated PID is that pockets of pus, or abscesses, can develop in the pelvic cavity. If these abscesses rupture, they spread infection in the pelvic cavity. This is called peritonitis. Peritonitis can be very dangerous and life threatening, similar to a ruptured appendix, and emergency surgery is necessary. The most serious results of PID (sterility, ectopic pregnancy, and major surgery) do not show up until five or ten years after the onset of the infection. Untreated PID can lead to scarring of the pelvic organs. If the tubes are scarred significantly, an egg will not be able to pass along the tubes and sterility results. The current risk of sterility after one PID episode is 20 percent.

Another aspect of scarring is that adhesions develop. Adhesions are internal scar tissue that, if they bind one organ to another, can cause pain. Adhesions can be removed surgically, but there is no guarantee they will not regrow.

Scarred tubes also increase the chances of an ectopic pregnancy. By the year 2000, 3 percent of women may have an ectopic pregnancy as a result of PID. Ectopic pregnancy is a pregnancy in which the egg is fertilized and implants in the fallopian tube rather than in the uterus. Ectopic pregnancies are very hazardous, since as the egg grows it becomes too large for the tube and the tube can suddenly rupture. The symptoms of acute PID are similar to the symptoms of ectopic pregnancy, so any sudden pelvic pain should be checked with a pregnancy test and other tests to rule out ectopic pregnancy.

If PID has not responded to other methods of treatment, or if abscesses have ruptured, a hysterectomy probably is necessary. But if you are under the care of a doctor, so that you know that you are not in severe danger, a program of self-healing could be very effective. Some infections can be self-limiting, so a program of extreme rest, careful avoidance of any foods to which you may be allergic, antibiotics as appropriate, and stress reduction activities can assist the body to heal its own infection. After all, an infection is the body's defense against unwanted bacteria. If you are able to assist your body in its own process of healing, you may have success.

Laura has a success story to tell.

> My PID was caused by an IUD, and in fact I am suing the manufacturers of the IUD for not informing my doctors of its risks. But I took the antibiotics, rested, and started a very restricted diet based on [Marshall] Mandell's book about allergies [*Dr. Mandell's Five-Day Allergy Relief System*]. So far I seem to be healing and I do not think I will need a hysterectomy.

Michelle's story is less cheerful.

> I think my hysterectomy was necessary, because I had been sick for a year by the time I had it. I got the pelvic infection and was treated with antibiotics. But I never really got better. First they did more antibiotics and hospitalized me for intravenous antibiotics and to do a laparoscopy. But nothing looked that bad so they didn't do any surgery until a few months later when I got worse again. Even then they took out only my tubes and one ovary. It wasn't until a year after the first infection that everything was removed. So I know the surgery was necessary, but I had a year of fever and constant pain. When I think of the cost for my life of that year, I really wonder whether it was best to delay the surgery, but I also wonder if I had started with rest and diet and the new styles of healing whether I could have avoided it altogether.

Rebecca had an experience common to women with PID.

> I went to the doctor and since I was black and female I think they must have thought I had gonorrhea before even testing me. They never did any tests but went ahead and put me on penicillin. My infection never cleared up, and

later they found out it wasn't a gonorrhea bacteria at all. I was really angry to be treated that way just because I was black. I have a friend who is white and middle class and they never even did a gonorrhea test on her because they "knew" she could not have gonorrhea.

PELVIC RELAXATION

Many hysterectomies, perhaps 14 to 29 percent, are done to correct pelvic relaxation or uterine prolapse. Usually occurring in a woman who has had several children, the condition involves weakening or relaxation of the muscles of the pelvic floor (that is, the area around the vaginal opening) or weakening or damage of the muscles or ligaments that hold the uterus in position in the pelvic cavity. Pelvic relaxation and prolapse are more common among white women than nonwhite women.

Symptoms of pelvic relaxation are a feeling of heaviness, pressure when bearing down to have a bowel movement, or the sensation that your "insides are falling out." This is due to the uterus dropping down into the vagina when it is no longer held in its normal place. When the condition is extreme, the uterus actually can protrude through the opening of the vagina, in fact turning itself "inside out." This condition is called uterine prolapse.

If you have uterine prolapse, you may also have cystocele or rectocele. Cystocele and rectocele are like hernias in the vagina. If the walls of the vagina become weaker, because of obstetrical intervention or a general lack of muscle tone, the bladder or rectum can bulge into the vagina. If you look again at the diagrams on pages 5 and 6, you will see that the organs are very close to the vagina. If it is the bladder (and urethra) that are bulging into the vagina, the condition is called cystocele or cysto-urethrocele; if it is the rectum that bulges into the vagina, it is called rectocele.

If you have either of these conditions, your bladder or your rectum may not function as well. If the angle of the bladder has changed, some urine may remain when you urinate. This will make you feel as though you still have to urinate even though you've just finished, and also may cause slight "leaks" when you cough or sneeze. Sometimes making a point of urinating in the bath or shower, and even having special shallow baths for this purpose, can help. That is normally an excellent method for treating cystitis and inflammation of the bladder, but with cystocele it could also help relax the bladder and urethra enough to completely empty the bladder. It is important to empty the bladder fully, particularly if you have cystocele, as you may be prone to frequent bladder infections. Drinking plenty of water, to flush out any bacteria that might collect, and emptying the bladder fully, especially in a warm bath or shower, are very helpful.

If it is the rectum that has ballooned into the vagina, constipation can result if the stool collects in the extra curves in the rectum. If this becomes a problem for you, you may find that increasing the bran in your diet, by introducing a teaspoon of miller's bran—plain, unprocessed bran—into your daily diet and increasing it to a half cup or so (gradually, or you may get severe cramps and diarrhea!) can help to keep your bowels moving. Many health professionals now believe that contemporary diets are deficient in roughage or fiber, and recommend that all of us increase our intake of bran.

A doctor can determine the kind of pelvic relaxation you have by asking you to "bear down" as if you were having a bowel movement while he or she is doing an internal examination. Some doctors also use a tenaculum, an instrument to grip the cervix, to check for prolapse. While you are lying down, the doctor can tug gently on the cervix and note where the uterus moves. This will give the information about what happens when you are standing up.

Good care of yourself at pregnancy and childbirth and good muscle tone in future years may help prevent pelvic relaxation. We should encourage ourselves and each other to keep our pelvic muscles firm by doing the Kegel exercise. This is tightening and relaxing the muscles in our pelvic floor. For most of us the best way to tell whether or not you're doing it is to pretend to or actually stop the flow of urine. The muscles we use to do this are the pelvic floor muscles, and we can exercise them any time of the day by tensing and relaxing them. If we do have weakening of the muscles, we may not be able to stop the flow of urine. Just as with any muscle, though, we can in fact rebuild the muscle tone by regular exercise.

If you have symptoms of uterine prolapse, spending time several times a day in the knee-chest position (that is, kneeling with your chest on the floor and your bottom in the air) can help to relieve them. What you do then is to let your organs slide back down into the pelvic cavity. If you are familiar with yoga exercises, the shoulder stand can be extremely relaxing and helpful for uterine prolapse.

Alternatives to hysterectomy for relieving the symptoms of pelvic relaxation include the use of a vaginal pessary and undergoing a suspension operation. A pessary is a device much like a diaphragm, which is left in place against the cervix in the upper end of the vagina. It holds the uterus up in place. It can cause irritation and discharge and can be uncomfortable, but if a short time using a pessary combined with Kegel exercises and yoga positions can prevent surgery, it could certainly be a good thing to start with. A suspension operation lifts and reattaches the uterus within the pelvic cavity.

Hysterectomy will cure uterine prolapse, since it removes the uterus, and at the same time the cystocele or rectocele can be repaired. Because of those repairs, hysterectomies for pelvic relaxation usually are done vaginally rather than through an abdominal incision.

Myra experienced a common assumption of doctors when she asked about a treatment for her prolapse.

I didn't realize until I got out of there what he had said. He said if they did the hysterectomy through the vagina they could tighten my vagina and my husband would like that. Now that I think of it I can't believe the nerve of that man.

Elizabeth eventually had a hysterectomy and is glad.

I didn't have any alternative doctors or anything but I did some exercising to try and get myself back in shape. I know maybe the hysterectomy was caused by mistakes around the time I had children, but there's nothing I can do about that now, and I'm not sorry it's all over.

Marian has used the prolapse as a signal to take better care of herself.

Around the time I was thirty-five I started having these problems and decided, well, forty is coming up and you'd better get yourself together. I read up on bowel trouble and bladder trouble and I started drinking more water and cranberry juice and eating more foods with fiber content. I started yoga too, and it's all been worth it. I feel much better. Forty is going to be a good year for me, and I still have my uterus.

ADENOMYOSIS

Adenomyosis is like a combination of endometriosis and fibroids. It is endometrial tissue that becomes embedded in the myometrium, the muscles of the uterus. Symptoms are heavy bleeding and a tender uterus. Diagnosis is difficult and one expert says it is the disease most often missed when present (and mistakenly thought to be fibroids) and most often diagnosed when not present. Final diagnosis is possible only after hysterectomy through pathological examination of the uterus. If a woman's symptoms are not severe, and a D & C (dilatation and curettage) has ruled out other problems, a "wait and see" approach is probably appropriate. Although 8 to 20 percent of hysterectomy patients are found to have adenomyosis, many have had hysterectomies for other reasons.

EXCESSIVE BLEEDING

Excessive bleeding is not a technical term and does not refer to any specific problem. But many of us have hysterectomies or have hysterectomies recommended to us when the doctors have no more explicit answer than that we have excessive bleeding. Excessive bleeding can cause weakness, making you less capable of regular activities during your period. It can also be a warning sign of serious problems. For example, excessive bleeding or irregular bleeding can be signs of uterine cancer. It certainly should not be ignored.

Another condition that could cause excessive bleeding is adenomyosis. This is the growth of endometrial tissue within the walls of the uterus. It makes the uterus tender and enlarged and can cause bleeding.

A first step in checking for the cause of excessive bleeding is often a D & C. D & C can be a method of abortion, although vacuum aspiration abortions have generally replaced it. It involves scraping the walls of the uterus so that the tissue removed can be checked for cancer or other abnormalities. Sometimes simply doing a D & C seems to cure the problem.

D & C is usually performed in the hospital, and often with a general anesthetic. If at all possible, try to avoid a general anesthetic, because the dangers from the anesthesia are far greater than the dangers from the D & C.

The dilation part of the D & C involves enlarging the opening of the uterus (dilating it) by inserting probes of increasing size through the cervix. One hazard of D & C is that the probe can accidentally puncture the uterus. As with all surgical procedures, it is important to choose the most skilled doctor you can. After the cervix is dilated, a curette, a metal loop on the end of a thin handle, is used to scrape the tissue from the walls of the uterus. Then the cervix is allowed to close.

During the recuperation time, ranging from a couple of hours to a couple of days, there may be some bleeding. This is normal, but any large clots or smelly discharge should be reported.

Evaluating the costs and benefits of having a D & C is similar to deciding about hysterectomy. D & C is far less hazardous than a hysterectomy and is an excellent method of checking for certain problems. On the other hand, any surgical procedure carries risks. Sometimes excessive bleeding is treated by repeated D & Cs, as often as one every year. Although this could make sense to avoid hysterectomy, repeated D & Cs carry their own risks too.

Unless you have reason to suspect you have a serious problem, you can try alternative ways of dealing with excessive bleeding before having D & C. Some recent research is suggesting that vitamin A may be very helpful for reducing heavy menstrual bleeding. The research showed that menorrhagia, heavy menstrual bleeding, may be caused by a vitamin A deficiency. The groups studied had been screened to rule out other problems, and they were found to have far lower vitamin A levels than women who had normal periods. When treated with vitamin A supplements each day, the women showed a definite improvement after one month. The amount of vitamin A recommended by the researchers is about 10,000 international units (IU) twice a day. They also suggest adding vitamin E and zinc. Vitamin E helps improve the body's use of vitamin A, as does zinc.

Norma Swenson, a member of the Boston Women's Health Book Collective who has done research and testimony on menopausal estrogens, notes a new "reason" for hysterectomy.

Many women in the premenopausal years experience irregular bleeding. Sometimes it is heavy bleeding, sometimes it is sudden, unpredictable gushes. It seems that one kind of menopause may be a heightened sensitivity, as in adolescence, to stress, dietary changes, exertion, emotional highs and lows, which is reflected in menstrual changes. Usually when this happens, a woman rushes to her doctor in panic and he usually suggests a D & C, "just to make sure."

What does this mean? It means that "he" wants to make sure the woman does not have some abnormality (e.g. cancer) and since cancer phobia is rampant she usually eagerly agrees. The D & C usually shows nothing, and for a month or two she is fine. But soon the bleeding returns. Another D & C. And now the soft, semi spongy lining of her uterus may even have been nicked or bruised by the curettage, so when the bleeding starts again, both she and her doctor are ready to say, "well, there really isn't any other approach. I could give you Provera for a while (that often doesn't work and has side effects) but why do you really need your uterus now anyway?" Enter hysterectomy. We in the book collective are convinced that it is worth the effort to either: avoid the first D & C, or at least the second, watch diet with extreme care and add Vitamin A, to see if the bleeding can be controlled. Eliminate alcohol, sugar, coffee, tea, etc.

Marjorie "waited to see" and has been able to postpone major surgery.

I decided to keep getting checked, but I was afraid of D & Cs. I read up on menopause and started a big health campaign. I don't know what did it, but the bleeding stopped. Here I am, past menopause and feeling terrific.

CANCER

Cancer is one of the most feared words in the language today. When we think cancer, we think death. But cancer is not death. It may feel like death, we may fear death, and some of us who have cancer will die. But cancer itself is not the same thing as death. If we let ourselves realize that, we may be less immobilized by our fear of death and more able to think clearly about cancer.

Only 8 to 12 percent of hysterectomies are due to cancer. Cancer means that a tumor or growth is malignant: that is, cells of that tumor or growth keep growing abnormally and can spread. The main dangers in cancer are that those cells can grow so rapidly that the organ being attacked is rendered useless. Also, cancer can spread to other parts of the body. Not all cancers do that. Particularly when you are older and your body is replacing cells more slowly and growing more slowly anyway, you can have a cancer that you live with for the rest of your life until you die of something else.

Cancer for which hysterectomy may be suggested can involve several parts of the body. It can be cancer of the cervix. The uterus can grow abnormal tumors in its body (cancer of the uterine corpus) or its lining (endometrial cancer.) Cancer of the ovary generally involves removing the uterus also, although there is some medical disagreement on this.

The American Cancer Society published the following statistics in 1978 on women in 1977 with gynecologic cancer.

GYNECOLOGIC CANCER 1977

SITES	NEW CASES	CANCER DEATHS
All female sites (inc. breast)	383,000	174,000
Invasive cervix	20,000	7,600
In situ cervix	40,000	—
Corpus of the uterus	27,000	3,300
Ovary	17,000	10,800
Other gynecologic	4,200	1,000

Cervical cancer, although more common, has a low death rate, and ovarian cancer, although there are many fewer cases, is much harder to treat satisfactorily. This is because cervical and uterine cancer frequently can be detected early.

The primary methods for detection of cancer in the pelvic area are the Pap test and attending to symptoms such as abnormal bleeding. Pap tests, named after Dr. George N. Papanicolaou, involve scraping cells from the cervical area inside the vagina. The scraping is done with a probe and can be momentarily uncomfortable. The cells are then analyzed in the laboratory, and the presence of abnormal cells is noted. Pap tests pick up cervical cancer, and regular Pap smears may have been responsible for early detection of many cancers and thus for saving many women's lives. At present there is a dispute, however, as to whether the decrease in cervical cancer deaths has been due to Pap tests or to nutritional and life-style changes. In addition, some analysts are debating whether annual Pap tests are cost-effective for the population. Perhaps the money is better spent on other prevention and treatment options.

Nevertheless, Pap tests are generally recommended each year, because cells can change and abnormal conditions can occur within a year. If a woman is "at risk" for cervical cancer, more frequent Pap smears are suggested. Being at risk for a condition or illness means there is reason to think you have a higher statistical likelihood of having that problem. For example, studies of large numbers of women have shown there is a higher rate of cervical cancer among women who became heterosexually active early in their lives, who had their first baby at a young age, and who have had many sexual partners. In addition, cervical cancer is more common in economically disadvantaged populations, and the incidence in black and Chicana women is double the incidence of cervical cancer in white women who live in the same geographic area. If you belong to those groups, it certainly does not mean you will get cervical cancer. Being "at risk" simply means you have a slightly higher probability of developing an illness than women who are not in those categories.

You would also be at risk if you have had suspicious cells on previous Pap tests, or if you know your mother took DES (diethylstilbestrol, a drug given to many pregnant women in the 1950s; see page 44.) In those cases you should plan more frequent Pap tests. Remember, even though you may be at risk, the chances are very, very strong you will not get cancer. You are simply being checked on somewhat more closely.

What happens if your doctor says you have suspicious cells on a Pap test? After you freak out and decide you are probably going to die tomorrow from cancer, you can clear your mind and settle down to think about what it means. Most people who have abnormal Pap tests do not have cancer. They usually have an infection that causes an abnormal reading on the tests. A Pap should be repeated two or three times to verify the information if it is suspicious.

You may be told you have dysplasia. Dysplasia simply means abnormal cells in the cervical area. Dysplasia does not mean cancer or that you are going to get cancer.

Traditionally, Pap smears have been classified as follows:

Type 1	Normal
Type 2	Atypical cells
Type 3	Suspicious cells
Type 4	Strongly suspicious for malignancy
Type 5	Conclusive for malignancy

Pap tests are known to have been inaccurate also. The tests are designed to have what statisticians call a bias toward false positive results. This means they try to be cautious in reporting the results to doctors so cases of cancer will not be missed. The result is that some women who have abnormal tests not only do not have cancer but do not have any abnormal cells at all. One study of 728 hysterectomies for cervical cancer estimates that incorrect diagnosis of Pap smears may have led to 150 unjustified hysterectomies.

Recent research has shown, though, that Pap tests do have a fairly high false negative rate. This means that 10 to 20 percent of Pap tests saying there are no abnormalities are wrong and the woman does have some abnormality. It is important to continue to have regular Pap tests, even if they are negative. Also, ask your doctor if the pathologist (the doctor who runs the laboratory where the tests are evaluated) has referred to the presence in the test of endocervical cells. Some doctors now think that if endocervical cells are not included in the Pap smear, the test may be invalid. It may well be that the first signs of cancer occur in the endocervical cells.

Most abnormal Pap smears are caused by chronic infection, chronic irritation of the cervix (cervicitis), or vaginal infection. To begin to check on your abnormal Pap smear the doctor looks at your cervix to see if there is a visible lesion. A lesion is an irritated or unusual-looking area. If there is no lesion, the chances are the doctor will prescribe a medicine, such as a vaginal cream, for infection and will suggest a second Pap test after the treatment is over.

If the doctor does see a lesion, the next step is to examine the abnormal area with a test called colposcopy. This involves careful checking for abnormal cells with a special, very powerful microscope. Frequently a staining technique is used with colposcopy to reveal the abnormal cells.

The next step is likely to be a biopsy, which means removing more cells than in the Pap smear and checking them under a microscope. The biopsy may be done in the doctor's office, or it may be necessary for you to go to the hospital overnight. The biopsy will probably show whether the lesion area is malignant or not. Most women who go to the hospital for a biopsy are found not to have a malignancy.

If cancer is found, it will be determined whether it is carcinoma in situ or invasive carcinoma. Carcinoma in situ means only one level of cells is affected. Invasive carcinoma has spread deeper into the cervical area.

It may be possible to remove the entire abnormal area with a procedure called conization. Conization involves removing a cone-shaped piece of tissue from the cervix. It is not a minimal or light procedure, as a major portion of tissue is removed. Conization should be done only if cancer is definitely discovered.

If you have carcinoma in situ, frequent colposcopy examinations to make sure it is not spreading may allow you to keep your uterus and, in fact, to have children.

Cervical cancer may be caused by a virus, perhaps the herpes virus that causes genital herpes and is related to the virus causing cold sores. Genital herpes is a very painful, recurrent vaginal condition. Recent research suggests that the herpes simplex 1 virus, the one causing cold sores, and the herpes simplex 2 virus, which causes genital herpes, may in fact be one virus, and women who have either cold sores or genital herpes should be checked carefully for signs of cervical cancer.

With other pelvic cancers there is no widely performed screening test like the Pap smear. It is very important to report any abnormal signs, because abnormalities and even cancers can be treated if identified early. Abnormal signs include abnormal bleeding and unusual pelvic pain. There are many, many causes for pelvic pain and abnormal bleeding. It continues to be worth checking even if you feel you are "bothering" the doctor, because these signs could mean a problem that could be stopped early.

Other pelvic cancers are actually very rare. Endometrial cancer, although definitely on the increase among women who have used estrogen drugs, nevertheless attacks very few women. It is most common in women who have already undergone menopause. Irregular bleeding is the most common symptom (*not* heavy periods), and a D & C is usually performed before a hysterectomy.

Cancer of the corpus (body) of the uterus is not common either, but it does tend to run in families. If you are overweight or diabetic, you should be especially careful to watch for abnormal bleeding.

As there is distinct evidence linking cancers of the uterus to estrogen drugs, it is a basic prevention strategy to avoid taking estrogen drugs.

Most women with cancer or precancerous conditions are not told of the option of delaying treatment to see if the cancer progresses. With regular checks, surgery frequently can be delayed, either until desired children have been born or sometimes indefinitely. Women often are rushed into surgery when they have not been fully emotionally prepared. A hysterectomy after your condition has been watched carefully for a period of months or even years will be far less terrifying because you will have done the emotional preparation. A hysterectomy three days after a positive Pap test leaves many women very frightened, and much of the emotional healing work cannot be done.

Ovarian cancer is even more rare, accounting for only about 1 percent of cancer cases in the population. Ovarian cancer is more common in women between forty and fifty years old, particularly those who are infertile or who have had ectopic pregnancies. When doctors say they should remove our ovaries before menopause to prevent ovarian cancer, we should remember the chances are very likely we will not get ovarian cancer even if our ovaries are left in.

Ovarian cancer is the hardest to detect, as it is less likely to produce bleeding or other discharge. Pay attention to pelvic pain, and encourage your doctor to examine you carefully. Although it is important for our doctors to be considerate and gentle with us, some doctors are too brief or superficial in their examination, so that women will not be caused discomfort and will return. It is important for the doctor during a checkup to feel each ovary and make sure it is not enlarged. This can be uncomfortable. Let yourself moan or say "ouch!" but encourage the doctor to check carefully. For overweight women in particular, the extra tissue plus the doctor's attitudes about obesity make checking the ovaries very crucial.

For confirmed cases of cancer there are generally three treatment-options within the medical model: surgery, radiation therapy, and chemotherapy.

Nonmedical alternatives for treatment of cancer can involve two major approaches. One is that the cancer or the tumor be "starved" by adopting a very restricted diet. This is the approach used by healers who follow natural hygiene principles. Other approaches involve mobilizing the person's will to live using visualization techniques and other treatments of the mind and the spirit.

The motivation of people to adopt self-healing methods with cancer is sometimes very high, because cancer is life-threatening. Seeking healers involved with cancer patients is also difficult, although increasing numbers of doctors are using a variety of approaches in dealing with cancer. Carl and Stephanie Simonton in Texas have regular programs to train people to use alternative approaches for treating cancer.

Women who have hysterectomies for cancer often have a different experience of the hysterectomy because it represents the saving of their life. Linda, for example, hardly thinks about the effects of the hysterectomy because she is so glad to be alive.

> I had had pain for quite a while—I was thirty-three—and I went in for cysts to be removed. When I woke up my husband's sweet voice was saying, "Linda, it wasn't cysts, it was malignant. They say it is terminal. Tell me you'll live." I told him, and I have lived. I use co-counseling to heal from the terror and rage I felt.

Edna, who is fifty years old, has not had a hysterectomy, although she has endometrial cancer.

You know, I don't think of it as being about saving my uterus. I think of it as trying to make myself healthy so this cancer will not grow anymore. My doctor doesn't do holistic medicine, but she is supportive of my crazy diet and spooky sessions as long as I keep coming to her for checkups. At my age, I'm really less concerned about the uterus than I am about saving my life, and I will have a hysterectomy if I have to. Right now I feel pretty good and pretty positive.

Nancy had cervical cancer and adopted the wait and see approach.

I was thirty-five, I had had a class 4 Pap smear for several years in a row, but I did not want a hysterectomy because I hadn't had children. I feel like I won a victory since my doctor "allowed me" to delay surgery. Finally I got pregnant, and my daughter was born. It was a very hard birth and when she was about nine months old I went ahead and had the hysterectomy. I think the hysterectomy is necessary at this point, but I'm glad I waited. She means everything to me.

We need to make sure we get the best medical diagnosis and treatment for our condition if we have cancer. We need to support alternative treatments for women's cancers, and to support women who choose or do not choose those approaches. But in addition we need to work to prevent cancer.

Probably 60 percent of the cancers in the United States today are triggered by environmental factors. We can work to prevent those cancers by helping to clean up pollution in the air, to discourage the use of pesticides for food and agriculture, to keep drugs out of the meat we eat, and to create safer work places. People working together *can* make a difference.

As individuals we can avoid toxic substances, in particular drugs, such as estrogen drugs, that are shown to be related to cancer. If we are currently taking birth control pills, we can use a different form of contraception. If we are taking estrogen drugs for menopause symptoms, we can try to cut down or detoxify our bodies from the drugs.

The healthier we are, the less likely we are to become ill, and the more likely we are to cope well with whatever illnesses we do get. This includes proper nutrition. Stop right now if you are about to feel guilty for having been sick! In our knowledge that we can take charge of our health and take better care of ourselves, we must never criticize ourselves if we are ill. We always do the best we can; it may be that becoming ill is the only way we can get the rest we need, or that working through the illness will be an important part of our personal growth.

Chapter Three

RATES and RISKS

Hysterectomy is now the most common major operation performed in the United States. The most recent, unpublished, data from the National Center for Health Statistics show that in 1979 over 640,000 American women had hysterectomies. Hysterectomy is now more common than tonsillectomy. Think about that. Since hysterectomies can be done only on women, that means every woman has a very high likelihood of having a hysterectomy during her lifetime.

Statisticians give varying projections of the hysterectomy rate. John Bunker, a doctor at Stanford University and expert on surgery rates, estimated that 50 percent of American women will have a hysterectomy by the age of 65 if present trends continue. Another estimate, published in the *American Journal of Obstetrics and Gynecology* in 1978, was that 62 percent of women in this country would eventually have a hysterectomy.

The number of hysterectomies performed in the United States

has been changing in the past decade or more. The Center for Disease Control recently analyzed the data collected by the National Center for Health Statistics for 1970 to 1975. The number of hysterectomies performed on women in the United States rose from 306,000 in 1970 to 430,000 in 1975, an increase of 40 percent. The rate of hysterectomies also increased, from 7.2 per 1,000 women fifteen to forty-four years of age in 1970 to 9.1 in 1975. Most of the increase occurred between 1970 and 1972, and after that, the rate remained nearly stable.

Recent data suggest the possibility of a slight reversal in the trend. The National Center for Health Statistics, which reported 640,000 hysterectomies in 1979, reported 705,000 in 1977, 678,000 in 1976, and 725,000 in 1975. One researcher reports a personal communication suggesting that a study by the Commission on Professional and Hospital Activities indicates a decline of 17 percent in the number of hysterectomies during the period 1975 to 1978. The major reason for any decrease in the rate of hysterectomy is heightened public and medical awareness of the number of hysterectomies that may not be necessary.

Despite any changes in the trends, the hysterectomy rate remains very high and many women have already had hysterectomies. One large study, published in 1980, was of women in the Seattle, Washington, area. The researchers found that one third of the women studied had had a hysterectomy already. Even among younger women, aged thirty-five to thirty-nine, 18 percent had already had a hysterectomy, and among women aged fifty-five to fifty-nine, 46 percent had already had a hysterectomy.

Hysterectomy is indeed an everyday event. More recently we have been hearing about unnecessary hysterectomy. What leads people to think many hysterectomies are unnecessary?

Twice as many hysterectomies are done on women with health insurance as on uninsured women. There also may be a variation in rate based on education and income. One study found higher income women had lower hysterectomy rates. Many more operations are performed if the doctor is paid on a fee-for-service basis than when the doctor is salaried, as in a prepaid group practice or in Great Britain. The hysterectomy rate can vary with the part of the country and sometimes with the part of the state.

The hysterectomy rate in one large teaching hospital rose 742 percent in a two and a half year period. It can vary with the time of year, rising when residency programs shift and the residents' "quota" of hysterectomies has not been met. The rate has been seen to drop dramatically in certain situations. When a health plan required all women who considered hysterectomy to have a second opinion, the number of operations performed dropped sharply. When a study of unnecessary surgery was announced in Saskatchewan, Canada, the hysterectomy rate in a period following the announcement dropped sharply.

Perhaps there are some genuine reasons for the increases in hysterectomy. We may be seeing genuine epidemics of some kinds of illnesses and therefore of some kinds of treatments. For example, there is a condition called adenosis, a precancerous condition of the vagina, which has been seen in daughters of women who took DES (diethylstilbestrol), a drug given to women in the 1950s in the mistaken hope that it might prevent miscarriage. It did not stop the miscarriages, and the children of the women who took DES now have previously unknown kinds of problems. Most DES daughters do not need hysterectomy, but some will.

Similarly, some hormone-related cancers are probably on the rise because of the large increase in the hormones we ingest in the form of birth control pills and hormones in the meat we eat. Estrogen replacement therapy (ERT) became extremely popular during the 1960s for women as young as thirty-five. One effect of taking estrogen drugs after menopause is unusual bleeding, which can be very alarming, as it can be a symptom of cancer. A woman experiencing unusual bleeding that could in fact have been caused by taking the estrogen drugs may have a hysterectomy. Estrogen drugs may stimulate fibroids and endometriosis, both common reasons for hysterectomy. So we may be seeing hysterectomies for conditions caused by estrogen drugs.

Increasing research may show a connection between some

kinds of cancer, as well as some women's diseases, and low-level radiation from nuclear power plants. Women working in certain occupations are known to have higher rates of reproductive disorders, such as miscarriages, infertility, or the birth of deformed children. Research is showing these reproductive disorders to be related to chemicals the women work with. It may be that some hysterectomies are caused by occupational or environmental factors.

Despite the undeniable fact that there are some new illnesses because of environmental, occupational, and chemical factors, the increase in hysterectomies cannot be explained by those reasons alone. Other factors do have an influence.

Women have made these observations in some of the workshops I have led:

Jane: I think they just want the money!

Tanya: You're not going to let them practice on me!

Gail: They told me it's saving lives by preventing cancer.

Sarah: I've heard that if you're in a group practice and you want a hysterectomy, sometimes it's hard to get one!

Carol: I'm a nurse, and the way those residents talk about women is just sickening. Once I heard a doctor say this hysterectomy was going to buy his Porsche.

These women all explain part of the picture. Jane is right. Financial motivation does play a role. We would not see so many more operations done by doctors paid for each operation (fee-for-service) than in situations where doctors are salaried, and therefore do not earn more for each procedure, if a financial interest were not at least subconsciously relevant. Some doctors openly acknowledge their financial motivation. One obstetrician/gynecologist was quoted in *The New York Times* as saying that since the birth rate is declining, "Some of us aren't making a living, so out comes a uterus or two each month to pay the rent," and others refer to a hysterectomy as "hip pocket surgery."

The number of women who tell stories of doctors' open greed is astonishing. At some level the profit motive is a very conscious part of current medical practice. Of course, it is easier to think about profit when you think of the body you are profiting from as being inferior, and in our society, women's bodies are seen that way. The profit motive in the medical field is coupled with the sexism basic to our society.

Most doctors do not consciously operate from a profit motive, and they generally try to have the best interests of women at heart. But in a society where "making it" is the most important goal and where "making it" is measured in dollars, where doctors have a very high social status and extremely high incomes, and where financial power and political power are closely linked, a profit motive is unconscious in any doctor working on a fee-for-service basis. It may never occur to us this way, but the private practice of medicine is one of the most lucrative small businesses around.

When Gail spoke of hysterectomies being done to prevent cancer, she is mentioning another major factor in the rise of hysterectomy rates. In the doctor's own words, many hysterectomies are done for "prophylactic" purposes. Ralph C. Wright, M.D., made one of the clearest statements of this: "The uterus has but one function: reproduction. After the last planned pregnancy, the uterus becomes a useless, bleeding, symptom-producing, potentially cancer-bearing organ and therefore should be removed."

Statistics do not support a preventive hysterectomy policy. Yet there is so much fear about cancer in the population, and so much concern in the medical profession to do whatever treatment might prevent a problem, that the risks and costs of the treatments themselves are often minimized.

PERSONAL DECISION: SOCIETAL RATE

Profit motive, the needs of teaching hospitals, and an underlying disregard for women's bodies are all parts of the explanation of high hysterectomy rates. Hysterectomy is a crucial personal decision for each woman, and all the personal decisions together add up to an important social phenomenon. Each woman needs to make her own decision and have her own relationship with her physician, but together all the individual decisions become rates.

In this country we tend to think of health care as an individual issue. We think of the costs of an operation, financial or physical, as costs only to the individual woman and her family. The true costs, however, are far broader. This point is easier to see in a country or situation where the receivers of health care share the costs, as in a national health plan like England's or in a prepaid health plan like Kaiser Permanente on the West Coast. In such arrangements any unnecessary health services cost all of the members in increased premiums or increased taxes. Even in this country we are aware of this relationship, because taxpayers can become very concerned about the high cost of providing health care to those people who cannot afford private health care services. The Reagan administration in 1981 proposed massive cuts in public health spending.

In fact, even in the fee-for-service health system all health care costs are borne indirectly by the whole society, and unnecessary surgery or unnecessary treatment costs are indirectly distributed to everyone. Money spent on unnecessary surgery, even if it is from the patient's own pocket, is money not spent on other goods and services that could be more useful to the economy. If a wealthy person should choose to have an unnecessary procedure, that may well mean that someone else less wealthy will not receive necessary care. In England doctors are shocked that in the United States the decision about surgery is up to the individual.

> In Britain, the health service rather than the patient is responsible for rationing and the broad selection of who shall have what. . . . However highly the British Health Service patient may judge the benefit to herself of elective hysterectomy, her chances of obtaining it are small when she has to compete with more demonstrably ill patients.

Because unnecessary surgery costs are costs to the entire economy, the Subcommittee on Oversights and Investigations of the U.S. House of Representatives held major hearings on unnecessary surgery in 1975 and 1977. In 1975 the subcommittee estimated that in 1974, 2,380,000 unnecessary operations were performed in the United States. Leading the list of operations often found unnecessary was hysterectomy. The dollar costs of these operations were $3.92 billion; the cost in avoidable deaths was estimated at 11,900 in 1974.

The money spent on drugs, treatments, and doctor bills from unnecessary surgery does profit someone. The concern of legislators and health activists is that the profits go to already wealthy individuals and already highly profitable industries, rather than to uses that society as a whole might choose.

For any of us, the decision certainly does not feel like it has to do with the entire society. We have a problem, and hysterectomy is suggested as a solution. None of us wants to think our hysterectomy was unnecessary.

Yet some of us do have unnecessary hysterectomies. Sometimes we do not have information on alternative treatments, sometimes we are severely alarmed by our physician's warnings, and sometimes we seek hysterectomy as a symbolic end to our childbearing years and a sign of freedom.

If you have had an unnecessary hysterectomy, *it is not your fault*. You were in a difficult situation, and you made the best decision you were able to make at the time. If today you see other options or other questions you could not hear at the time, that means today something is different in your life.

RATES OF UNNECESSARY SURGERY

Few doctors or policy analysts will define necessary and unnecessary hysterectomy. Individual differences and the high degree of subtlety in medical options make clear definitions impossible. Most analysts find it useful to look at rates and large numbers. They will cautiously define indications for hysterectomy they consider truly unnecessary, but generally they prefer to examine rates, and the way the rates vary, to determine the proportion of unnecessary surgery.

Attention is generally drawn to rates of surgery when those rates change dramatically or are seen to vary with factors that are not strictly medical. Then policymakers go about determining more accurately the actual number of hysterectomies that might have been unnecessary.

One method for estimating rates of unnecessary surgery is the use of preset criteria. A panel of doctors prepares a list of acceptable reasons for hysterectomy. Then someone takes a stack of patient records of hysterectomies performed, perhaps all the records from a particular hospital or a sample of records from all the procedures done in a particular state or health plan. The worker then compares these records with the criteria outlined by the panel of experts. The number of unnecessary procedures is the number of cases in which the criteria were not met.

By the standards of health activists studies using this method define unnecessary procedure very cautiously. Dr. Frank Dyck, who led one of the major studies using this method, said, "We were deliberately liberal so we would have credibility with the doctors. We considered hysterectomies unjustified only if they were prophylactic or 'birthday' hysterectomies, when a woman turned forty, or if they were based on 'surgical clairvoyance.' "

The list of indications prepared by Dr. Dyck's expert committee in Saskatchewan included:

Malignant conditions
Premalignant conditions
Endometriosis
Large fibroids
Severe infections
Benign tumors
Unusual bleeding
Pelvic congestion syndrome (a controversial category including symptoms such as low back pain and menstrual pain)

The only indications clearly unnecessary in the Saskatchewan study were hysterectomies for the purpose of sterilization or prevention of cancer where there was no reason to suspect cancer. Some doctors, however, would not suggest hysterectomy for endometriosis, fibroids, or menstrual pain unless these were very severe.

The study was done by the Saskatchewan Department of Health after they noticed the number of hysterectomies in their province had jumped by 72.1 percent between 1964 and 1971, while the number of women over fifteen years of age increased by only 7.6 percent. When the charts of five hospitals were sorted using the criteria described above, the number of unnecessary hysterectomies ranged from 17 percent to 59 percent of the hysterectomies performed.

The Saskatchewan study had an unanticipated side effect. When the study was announced, the hysterectomy rate dropped sharply, probably because hospitals began using more careful review and documentation procedures. However, it appears that within five years hysterectomy rates had returned to close to the previous levels.

Another way to estimate the numbers of unnecessary procedures (and to reduce those numbers) is second-opinion programs. Some health plans or insurers, such as the Teamsters union health plan in New York City, have introduced either voluntary or mandatory second opinions for women whose first physician suggests hysterectomy. The second-opinion programs work in one of two ways. If the program is voluntary, the plan will pay for a second opinion on the request of the woman. If the plan has mandatory second opinions, the woman is required to have the concurrence of a second physician before the plan will pay for her hysterectomy. The rationale of the health plans is that the cost of the additional doctor visit will be offset by savings in avoiding higher-cost surgery, although this is more recently in dispute.

In one study of the second-opinion program the second physician did not confirm the first physician's recommendation of hysterectomy in 43 percent of those second opinions requested by the woman. The mandatory second opinion did not concur with the first recommendation in 21 percent of the cases. That discrepancy is predictable, because if the second opinion is voluntary, second opinions will be requested primarily by those women who have some doubt about the recommendation of the first doctor. When the second-opinion program is required for everyone, the numbers include those women whose hysterectomies are definitely necessary, causing the percentage of second opinions that do not agree to drop.

Critics of this study say the percentages do not indicate unnecessary procedures: perhaps the second doctor is incorrect and the hysterectomy is necessary. However, after one to five years, more than 80 percent of those women who had a second opinion that did not confirm the first recommendation for surgery did not in fact have the hysterectomy.

Today many policy experts agree on the high rate of unnecessary hysterectomy. They differ on the way to reduce those rates. The California State Assembly held hearings on unnecessary hysterectomy in November 1979. At those hearings the representative from the trial lawyers' organization thought the best method to reduce unnecessary hysterectomy was malpractice suits. Representatives from Blue Cross thought there should be some prior review by Blue Cross staff before elective surgery but there should be no mandatory second opinion. Representatives from the Professional Standards Review Organization (PSRO) said in fact they were reviewing and monitoring unnecessary surgery. Representatives from the California Medical Association said that informal peer review by physicians was the best method of reducing unnecessary surgery.

No one was invited to represent consumers at those hearings. Each group declared itself to be the most effective agent to reduce unnecessary surgery. But none of the methods described is fully effective. Malpractice insurance has contributed to the enormous increase in the cost of medical services, and most malpractice cases are brought because of a doctor's failing to perform a treatment, rather than his performing an unnecessary treatment. A review panel hired by Blue Cross to screen proposed operations is far less costly, and far less effective, than a second-opinion program. PSROs are notoriously ineffective, and peer review is widely thought to be an unsatisfactory method of supervising the work of physicians.

The most effective methods of reducing the rate of unnecessary surgery are based in public action. Public pressure, media attention, and government hearings bring about an increased awareness, setting the stage for legislative or regulatory actions that can affect surgery rates. For example, in response to research, public awareness, and lawsuits about the high rate of sterilization by hysterectomy, federal guidelines in 1978 prohibited that practice. However, widespread noncompliance with the guidelines is reported.

ELECTIVE HYSTERECTOMY

In general, defenders of high hysterectomy rates recommend hysterectomy for two reasons that are not on the "necessary" list of most groups reviewing rates. They recommend elective hysterectomy for the purpose of sterilization, and prophylactic hysterectomy to prevent possible future diseases such as cancer. A hysterectomy for either of these reasons is not medically indicated and will not cure an existing medical problem.

Of course, decisions are made for many reasons, and some "unnecessary" hysterectomies do meet women's needs as they perceive them. For example, women for many years have used hysterectomy as a subterfuge if for religious reasons they could not use contraception. A hysterectomy for "female troubles" would relieve them of the need to use contraception while not challenging their religious beliefs.

Some women willfully choose to end their childbearing capacity by a sterilization operation. The most common method today is tubal ligation: that is, the cutting or tying or burning of the fallopian tubes, which prevents eggs from passing into the uterus. After tubal ligation, a woman will continue to have periods, but simply cannot get pregnant. The easiest method of tubal ligation these days is called the laparoscopic method. Only a very small incision needs to be made in the abdomen, and the procedure can be done with a minimum of anesthesia. Tubal ligation itself is increasingly under scrutiny. Many women report heavy bleeding or menstrual pain, and studies have shown that women who had laparoscopic sterilization have an increased likelihood of hysterectomy. Health activists are recommending other forms of contraception, such as diaphragms, cervical caps, or foam and condoms, rather than sterilization.

Hysterectomy is virtually never a rational alternative to tubal ligation. Compared to tubal ligation, hysterectomy costs four to five times more, has a complication rate ten to twenty-two times higher, and a death rate of 300 to 500 per 100,000 compared to 14 to 22 per 100,000 for tubal ligation. Yet hysterectomy is frequently performed for sterilization.

The other reason for elective hysterectomy is to prevent disease, primarily uterine or ovarian cancer. Some might argue that for the society as a whole it would make sense to give women hysterectomies to prevent future cancers. After all, the costs for treatment and surgery for cancer are high when added together. In addition, hysterectomy for all women would save the country certain costs. Less would be spent on menstrual products like Kotex or Tampax. Also, fewer children would be born with Down's syndrome, since that happens generally to women over the age of thirty-five. Perhaps it would make sense to remove this unnecessary organ from all women at the age of thirty-five in order to save society these costs.

Following the suggestion of proponents of elective hysterectomy, Philip Cole and Joyce Berlin of Harvard University calculated the costs and benefits of removing every woman's uterus when she reached thirty-five, and published their results in the *American Journal of Obstetrics and Gynecology* in 1977. Even with this "coldly rational" analysis, hysterectomy to prevent cancer did not make economic sense. The costs in dollars turned out to be higher if unnecessary surgery was done than the costs of treating uterine cancer. In addition, the years of life gained when spread over the entire population were very small.

Yet this approach has been recommended by a number of prominent physicians. James H. Sammons, executive vice-president of the American Medical Association, testified in 1976 before a House subcommittee that women should have hysterectomies if they are anxious about getting cancer or if they wish sterilization.

Ralph C. Wright's classic statement points to the following benefits of elective hysterectomy after the last planned pregnancy:

1. The nuisance, inconvenience, and disability of menstrual periods are eliminated.

2.   Pain and discomfort associated with menstruation are no longer a problem.

3.   As a sterilizing operation, the need for prolonged use of contraceptives no longer exists. Fear of pregnancy is no longer disturbing. The tragedy of an unwanted pregnancy late in menstrual life is eliminated.

4.   Hospitalization for curettage and conization of the cervix is no longer necessary.

5.   There is no longer a need for the annual cytologic smear [Pap smear].

6.   Fear of cancer of the uterus is eliminated; loss of life from cancer of this organ is now of no concern.

7.   If, in addition, both ovaries are removed, further benefits accrue. Replacement therapy is simple and inexpensive. Premenstrual tension is no longer a problem. Another common source of inoperable malignancy is eliminated.

In summary, elective hysterectomy is prophylactic and sterilizing and provides permanent symptomatic relief. The patient can now lead a happier and more comfortable and productive life, free from the anxieties and the monthly problems associated with the useless and potentially lethal reproductive organs.

Many American obstetricians and gynecologists strongly support the positions of doctors Wright and Sammons. At its 1971 annual meeting held in San Francisco, the American College of Obstetrics and Gynecology sponsored what is now fondly remembered as the "Great Debate" on the merits of hysterilization. Following the exchange, physicians were asked to register their approval or disapproval of this procedure by their applause. The acclaim for hysterilization lasted a full twenty-five seconds: the applause for the "no" position, only ten seconds. What's more, according to *Audio-Digest's* Decibel Meter, the intensity of the advocates' applause was double that of the opposition.

Proponents of elective hysterectomy point to the fact that uterine and ovarian cancer kill women each year. That is undeniably true. But so do unnecessary hysterectomies. In fact, the deaths from uterine cancer in a year are about the same as the death from unnecessary hysterectomy, and uterine cancer is often preventable with good Pap tests. Also, the American Cancer Society estimates that in 1977 in the U.S. nearly 60,000 men developed prostate cancer and 20,000 died. They estimated the same number of women developed cervical cancer, and 7,600 died. Statistically it would make more sense to remove the prostate to prevent cancer, yet that is virtually never mentioned.

If a woman could truly predict with some degree of accuracy that she might have uterine or ovarian cancer, then hysterectomy could be a rational alternative. But no one can predict this. Regular checkups reveal uterine or cervical cancer generally in early enough stages that they can be treated. Choosing to have a hysterectomy means undergoing a real risk of illness or death within the next year, while uterine cancer is a possible outcome at some time in the future. Most of the risk from hysterectomy is from anesthesia. It appears preferable to entertain a possible future risk rather than undergo a present definite risk. Your personal decision must be based on your personal predictions of the risks and benefits of surgery.

Those of us who speak out against unnecessary surgery are making a difference. One estimate is that the rate of hysterectomy has gone down 17 percent. Of course, fewer women are available for a hysterectomy if many have their uteruses removed each year.

But many of us speaking out, in small voices to our doctors, in amplified voices through the media or our lawyers, and in policymakers' voices through our representatives, have made a difference. Sometimes we feel very powerless when we look at the enormity of the problem. But any problem is more likely to be solved by numbers of people working together in many small ways. We have a long way to go before women will be totally in charge of what happens to their bodies. But we are making some headway.

REAL RISKS

Many of us are fortunate enough to feel better after hysterectomy. Most of us do not have major complications with the surgery. The fear of complications should not keep us from having an operation that is truly advisable. But knowledge of possible complications and aftereffects can help us weigh risks and benefits of the surgery and also encourage us to report symptoms more promptly and firmly.

The death rate, 0.3 to 0.5 percent, is lower than that for some other operations, but far higher than that for nonsurgical or less extensive procedures. The rate of complications is 30 to 40 percent and includes problems ranging from minor urinary-tract infections to thromboembolism or permanent damage to the bladder or ureter.

Infection—of the incision area or of the bladder—is not uncommon and generally is treated by antibiotics. Hemorrhage is much less common, as is accidental cutting of the rectum, bladder, or ureter. Incidentally, the likelihood of these surgical accidents seems to be related to the skill and experience of the surgeon. It probably makes sense to have the most skilled surgeon you can find do the actual operation, even if your personal doctor follows you and gives better, more supportive, health care. Most of us, however, are not in a position to judge this.

Any anesthesia carries major risks, of allergic reaction or heart or lung complications, and it is important to cooperate with the health team in the history-taking and postoperative exercises to help prevent problems. Nerve trauma sometimes occurs and leads to weakness or sometimes permanent damage to the nerves.

Hormone levels may be affected, at least temporarily, by hysterectomy even if the ovaries are left in. This could be the reason many women have hot flashes and unusual fatigue after this particular operation.

Urinary problems after hysterectomy are very common and range in severity from minor to serious. They can result from infection of the bladder from the catheter, trauma or damage to the bladder or ureter or urethra, or accidental cutting of the urinary organs. Note in the diagrams on pages 5, 6, and 7 how close together these pelvic organs are.

After surgery some women develop adhesions, internal scar tissue that forms weblike bands that can bind various pelvic structures together. Adhesions are more common after surgery involving infection. They can range from unnoticeable, to those causing some occasional pain if they bind, for example, the end of the vagina to part of the bowel, to those that are very serious if they eventually obstruct the bowel.

Some studies indicate that many women gain weight after hysterectomy. It is unclear whether this is a result of metabolic changes, psychological distress, social expectations, or a combination. If a woman is concerned about gaining weight, she should try to consider whether in fact it is rational for her to try to avoid it. We have such strong societal messages telling us to be very thin that it is hard to be clear about whether a weight gain is in fact a problem. But we should be aware that others have gained weight after hysterectomy.

If the ovaries are removed, additional problems can occur. The effects of "menostop" can be very distressing. A woman considering ovariectomy should know that if she has not already finished menopause she will probably notice major changes, which diminish as her body adjusts to the new hormone level.

Ovariectomy causes so-called minor changes in body hair, skin tone, and body fat, and it may lead to more frequent vaginal infections. After ovariectomy estrogen drugs are generally prescribed. Women are thus required to make difficult decisions about relief from symptoms versus the risk of taking a potentially dangerous drug. Risks of estrogen replacement therapy include gallbladder trouble, thromboembolism, a possible effect on glucose tolerance, and perhaps a connection with breast cancer, although the research in this area is conflicting. Ironically, estrogen replacement therapy may cause bleeding which can lead to hysterectomy. Also, *discontinuing* the estrogen can lead to osteoporosis.

COMPARISONS WITH OTHER PROCEDURES

As major operations go, hysterectomy is very safe. It is more dangerous to have surgery in areas higher up the body cavity. That is, heart surgery and certainly brain surgery are far more hazardous than pelvic surgery. Medical advances in preventing infection by using antibiotics before the operation have made a big difference in the safety of the procedure. Additionally, advances in the technology of anesthesia have improved life-chances with hysterectomy. So it is safer to have a hysterectomy than to have brain surgery. But that is not the situation most women find themselves in. They are comparing hysterectomy with other alternatives for the condition that they have.

Hysterectomy is far more hazardous than tubal ligation, if a woman wants to end her childbearing capacity. Hysterectomy is far more hazardous than bed rest and a dict change, if that treatment is available for her problem. In fact, the risks of hysterectomy must be compared with the actual alternatives a woman faces.

To help put the risks of hysterectomy in perspective, research-ers have compared outcomes of hysterectomy with other, similar surgery. The most common comparison is gallbladder surgery, because the gallbladder is also in the pelvic cavity. In comparison with gallbladder surgery, hysterectomy carries statistically greater risks. More women have psychological problems after hysterectomy than after a gallbladder operation. The likelihood of dying after hysterectomy is higher than the likelihood of dying after gallbladder surgery.

It is true that the risks of death following unnecessary hysterectomy are less than the risks of death following necessary hysterectomy. That is, more women who have a hysterectomy with no previous medical problem will survive that hysterectomy than those women that have a hysterectomy because of a previous medical problem. That statistic is sometimes used to show how safe unnecessary or elective hysterectomy is. But of course a woman who has a hysterectomy because of severe infection or because of cancer is unwell to begin with. Her chances of dying are higher than those of a woman in excellent health. The comparison should be between hysterectomy and not having a hysterectomy when there is no medical reason.

PERSPECTIVE

The rates of hysterectomy reflect trends in the United States medical system, trends toward more surgery, particularly in situations where there is profit, and on women and minority group members. On the other hand, some individual women find themselves with a problem for which hysterectomy appears to be the only solution, and fewer women who have hysterectomies will die from them today than at times in the past. Each woman needs to make her own decision based on her own best calculation of her risks and her benefits. At the same time we can work to change the trends so that there will be fewer hysterectomies in the society as a whole.

We can work on this on all fronts. We can become more assertive health care consumers and more alert nurses and doctors, we can support government efforts to reduce surgery abuse, and we can remind ourselves that we make the best decisions we can.

Chapter Four

WAR on the WOMB

When we look at hysterectomy rates and at the way ideas about women have influenced our health care system, we see the trend toward more hysterectomies in a different light.

ELECTIVE HYSTERECTOMY AS A MEDICAL CRIME AGAINST WOMEN

Elective hysterectomy (hysterectomy that is not necessary medically) may be done for sterilization, or it may be done to prevent cancer. Medically, the rationale for hysterectomy in both of these situations is very weak. Yet elective hysterectomy is vigorously supported by many doctors.

Suppose we think of unnecessary hysterectomy as a crime. We can call it a crime because it involves unnecessary mutilation, and it involves subjecting a woman to unnecessary risks. It represents one person profiting from the risky mutilation of another. We do, after all, generally consider it a crime if one person wounds another for money.

Today we hear more and more about "white-collar crime," and we are more likely to compare corporate actions to crimes. For example, some refer to the practices of big business as "crimes in the suites." Cynicism about the medical profession is also growing, and I hear increasing numbers of women speaking of unnecessary surgery as a crime.

Unnecessary hysterectomy is also often a con job. The person may come in wanting to be sterilized or concerned about cancer. To present hysterectomy as the only possible option certainly smacks of a con job.

Diana Scully, who has done extensive research on the sources of medical attitudes toward hysterectomy, describes the "bait and switch" tactic used by doctors to talk women into hysterectomy. The bait is sterilization by tubal ligation. Residents (doctors in training for a specialty, who actually perform many operations, especially on clinic patients) used a standard strategy to talk women who had come requesting tubal ligation into hysterectomy.

> The sales pitch used by residents at both hospitals was remarkably similar; in some cases the very same words were used. The resident opened by moving from a general problem for which a number of solutions, including doing nothing, were possible, to the solution he was going to try to sell, usually a hysterectomy. The more supporting evidence that could be brought to bear on the problem, the more secure the resident was in his pitch. The pitch frequently began when a woman over the age of thirty-five requested birth control or permanent sterilization in the form of a tubal ligation. If, in addition, the resident could locate evidence of some pathology, he would attempt to sell a hysterectomy. Essentially, the resident was substituting a hysterectomy (surgery he wanted to do) for a tubal liga-

tion (surgical scut work). The tactic was similar to the "bait and switch" technique used in sales in which the advertised item is discredited and another, more expensive, product is substituted in its place.

These parallels between unnecessary hysterectomy and crime or sharp business practice help us to see the medical system in a new light. After all, health care is one of the biggest industries in this country today, and the private practice of medicine is one of the most profitable small businesses around. We should not be surprised that a medical system so profitable could lead to abuses. The problem, of course, is that the consumer can be victimized physically as well as financially.

We should remember that many crimes against women are more socially acceptable than similar acts against men would be. For example, rape is a crime against women that only recently has been treated seriously. Rape victims themselves have often felt as if they were criminals.

Wife abuse or woman battering include acts that are assault and criminal acts if they take place in a context other than a domestic situation with a woman as victim.

Uncomfortable though it may be, we need to realize that many crimes against women are socially acceptable, or at least have been socially acceptable. If unnecessary hysterectomy is a medical crime, the fact that it is uniquely a crime against women contributes to its acceptance by all of us as well as to its invisibility.

SEXISM AND MEDICAL IDEOLOGY

Most doctors do not perceive themselves to be criminally abusing women for profit. In addition, most women do not see themselves as victims of crimes. But sexism is so deeply rooted in medical ideology, and medical "science" is so instrumental in the systematic suppression of women, that medical crimes against women are taken for granted.

We can see the relationship more clearly if we look back one hundred years. In the eyes of nineteenth-century medical theory women were sick. Puberty, menopause, pregnancy, menstruation, all aspects of a woman's life cycle, were pathological. Women needed medical care for these problems. Generally the cures were enforced rest and other, more hazardous procedures.

It was also one hundred years ago that women were beginning to question their role and move out of some of the traditional expectations. However, the medical requirement of bed rest for nearly every female experience effectively kept women from organizing.

Dr. Frederick Hollick, author of a well-known book of 1850, asserted that menstruation

> . . . makes it impossible for woman, except in a few peculiar individual cases, to pursue the same mode of life as men. It makes her, of necessity, not so continuously active, nor so capable of physical toil, while, at the same time, it causes her to yearn for sympathy and support from some being that she feels is more powerful than herself.

Women doctors saw through this, and the president of Bryn Mawr College wanted a female doctor for her students. "She will prescribe sheer idleness as a remedy neither for the indisposition of girls in their teens, nor for the ill health of college students."

A famous medical theory of the 1800s postulated a relationship between the reproductive and mental organs. Overuse of one area was thought to lead to atrophy of the other. For men this led to cautions against excessive sexual activity, which could inhibit mental functioning. For women, however, mental activity was thought to stunt reproductive activities. The implication, a belief championed by President Theodore Roosevelt and supported by medical experts of the time, was that higher education would destroy the reproductive abilities of American women.

For all of the problems women have, constant medical attention was necessary. In the 1800s medical doctors as we know them today were only a sect competing with other kinds of healing. Part of the strategy of building the popularity of the profession of medicine was creating many illnesses that only doctors could cure.

The treatments for female complaints included bed rest and leeches and chemicals applied to the vulva and drugs such as heavy doses of opium. But women of the 1800s were also subjects of new surgical techniques. One controversial but frequently performed operation was to remove the clitoris. Gena Corea documents the promotion of the clitoridectomy not only as a treatment for masturbation, but also as a treatment for

> indigestion, insomnia, fissure of rectum, pain in back or side, sterility, an inability to look one straight in the face, painful urination, melancholy, headache, a desire to run away from home or to become a nurse, heart palpitation, anemia, swollen joints, failing eyesight, dry skin, and clammy skin.

Historian G. J. Barker-Benfield studied the uses of gynecological surgery in the 1800s and found ovariectomy especially frequently used. Among the indications for ovariectomy were "troublesomeness, eating like a ploughman, masturbation, attempted suicide, erotic tendencies, persecution mania, simple internal 'cussedness' and dysmenorrhea." Most apparent in the enormous variety of symptoms doctors took to indicate castration was strong sexual appetites in women.

How much more clearly can scientific ideology as a way of keeping women less powerful be expressed? It is ironic that ovariectomy, promoted one hundred years ago as a cure for excessive sexuality, today is frequently accompanied by the assurance that there will be no change in sexuality after ovariectomy.

It was only the middle-class women, who could afford them, who "benefited" from the new medical treatments. Working-class women, who experienced an actual rate of tuberculosis, malnutrition, and other serious disease far higher than middle-class women, were considered hearty enough to work long hours without benefit of medical care, even in childbirth.

But that was one hundred years ago. Today medical ideas are much more modern, and today science is objective, we say. Are things really so very different today? Let us think about medical ideology as it affects women. We are aware that Valium is the most highly prescribed drug in the world, and most of the prescriptions for this mood-altering, frequently unnecessary drug are for women. We're aware there remains no safe and effective commonly used form of birth control. We are aware that life changes during menopause are very frequently treated as an illness that requires a dangerous hormone drug. We are aware that childbirth is increasingly a medical experience, with high use of drugs and surgery. And hysterectomy, the commonest major operation today, is a woman's operation. Medical ideas, theories, and treatments continue to affect women's roles on many levels.

MEDICINE AND SOCIAL CONTROL

Irving Kenneth Zola, a sociologist from Brandeis University, first developed the idea of medicine as a system of social control. Barbara Ehrenreich, John Ehrenreich, and Deirdre English have continued to develop those ideas, which are extremely important in understanding women's experiences.

Generally we think of social control as the "negative" forces in our society. We think of the police or the criminal justice system as social control. In fact, any social system has social controls. Social control is not necessarily positive or negative. It includes all the ways a society "keeps people in line" or gets people to do the appropriate things. Social control includes the education system, social service system, and even the health system. It includes all the ways we get messages about what we should or should not do.

Medicine is a system of social control because it reflects the American social system. The people with most authority, doctors, tend to be white, wealthy, and male. Women's role in the medical system reflects women's role in the larger society. Women are nurturers, nurses, and are seldom in decision-making positions. Minority group members, children, the elderly, the disabled, and the poor have especially powerless positions in the health system. This reflects their positions in the larger society.

As well as reflecting the social structure, the medical system reinforces the relationships of the larger social system. When we enter a relationship with a doctor, it is one of intimacy, but it is one-way intimacy. We are expected to reveal parts of our bodies and parts of our lives to the doctor. The intimacy is not reciprocal: we call the doctor "Dr. X," and the doctor frequently calls us by our first name or "dear." The doctor seldom shares personal facts.

The doctor–patient relationship reinforces, in very subtle and subconscious ways, the assumption that it is white upper-class males who appropriately hold power over us. We need not look too far to see more examples of medicine as social control. It is doctors who offer relief from physical or psychological pain, and it is doctors who let us know what is normal. It is doctors who determine if you are fit to work, or if your children would suffer and therefore you must not work. It is doctors who prescribe mood-altering drugs instead of encouraging us to change our lives. It is doctors who promote sterilization for some groups, and who make abortion unavailable for other people.

There is nothing wrong with health care being social control. In a society with a different political structure or a different dominant ideology, health care would reflect and reinforce those structures and ideologies. When we point to problems in the medical system, generally we are pointing to problems that are characteristic of the entire society. Conversely, the gains we make in the women's health movement in providing alternative models of care and promoting a more active role for women make an impact on society in general as well as on the health care system.

HYSTERECTOMY AND SOCIAL CONTROL

Hysterectomy has a key role in the social control of women. Minority group women are in many ways the least powerful adults in society. Hysterectomy has been so common among black women in the South that it has been referred to as "Mississippi appendectomy." Women experience the threat of hysterectomy and/or sterilization if they seek an abortion. There are many documented accounts of women on welfare having been told that welfare payments would not continue unless they were sterilized or had a hysterectomy. This is not legal, and probably is less common practice today than it has been in the past. The concerted action of minority group women has resulted in changes in some of the more obvious abuses.

Many women of minority groups are poor, and the health care they receive is often in public hospitals or teaching hospitals. The doctors in teaching hospitals are under pressure to perform a certain number of hysterectomies for their teaching experience. Frequently minority group women are victims of doctors pressuring them into surgical procedures they may not want. At the Los Angeles County–University of Southern California Medical Center during a two-and-a-half-year period in the late 1960s, the increase in the number of hysterectomies performed was 742 percent. The number of elective hysterectomies specifically for sterilization increased by 293 percent. In recent years the number of hysterectomies performed on white women has been increasing rapidly, but still a higher proportion of black women have hysterectomies than white women.

Sterilization abuse is any active or de facto restriction of a woman's right to choose to bear or not to bear children. Sterilization abuse includes procedures performed without consent or when consent is under duress, when a woman is led to believe that sterilization is reversible, when sterilization is the condition for abortion or welfare benefits, when sterilization is done for "eugenic purposes," is falsely presented as safe or "medically indicated," or when a person truly chooses sterilization but is denied the operation.

CARASA, the Committee for Abortion Rights and Against Sterilization Abuse, suggests that sterilization abuse is a major problem among minority and poor women, and it presents some disturbing facts suggesting that there may be a deliberate policy by government and family planning agencies to sterilize minority group members. CARASA cites a 1978 study of federal figures that shows an increase of sterilization among low-income women in the age group twenty-five to thirty-four. Among low-income white married women in the U.S. in 1976, 37 percent had been sterilized, an increase of 11 percent from 1973. Among black low-income married women in the age group twenty-five to thirty-four, sterilizations increased from 16 to 24 percent. In contrast, for higher-income women the increase in sterilization rate is among women over thirty-five years old, that is, those who are more likely to have already completed their families. A confirmed 35.3 percent of all women of childbearing age in Puerto Rico, and perhaps as many as 25 percent of all native American women, have been sterilized, many of them involuntarily. Sterilization of minority women is more common in certain areas, and a study in New York City found that twice as many black and six times as many Hispanic women as white women are sterilized in municipal hospitals.

Hysterectomies are not necessarily included in these figures. The number of women sterilized by hysterectomy for possibly flimsy medical reasons other than sterilization is higher. More black women than white women are sterilized, but the numbers are very high when all sterilizations, including hysterectomy for "medical" reasons, are included.

	Percentage
White married women	17.8
Black married women	19.7
White unmarried women	29.9
Black unmarried women	30.4

Perhaps the high percentage of minority and low-income women who are sterilized represents many individual decisions for sterilization. But the policy toward funding of abortion and sterilization shows a disturbing relationship. Even without the so-called human life amendment, federal, state, and local funding for abortion has been cut off in most areas. Yet the federal government still assumes 90 percent of the cost of sterilization operations under Medicaid. U.S. policy in third-world countries is openly one of encouraging sterilization. It appears possible that those policies are applied to low-income and minority women in the United States as well.

Some changes are taking place. Probably because of the efforts individually and in concert of minority group women and their supporters, the rates of sterilizations have leveled off and the rates of hysterectomy among black women have not significantly increased. In 1978 the Department of Health, Education and Welfare issued guidelines regulating federally funded sterilizations. The guidelines require informed consent in the person's preferred language. Unfortunately, several investigations have shown the weakness in enforcing these guidelines. The changing political climate of the 1980s, with increased visibility of anti-abortion, antiwomen groups and weakening of federal regulatory agencies in nearly every area, is likely to provide a climate for new growth in sterilization abuse.

For minority group women hysterectomy rates have an impact on the future of the minority of which they are members as well as on them as individuals. They experience racism in the doctor/patient relationship, often without the well-meaning health worker's perception that racism is involved.

Important as this analysis is at the societal level, we come back always to the experience of women. What is a hysterectomy decision like for women of color, also called third-world women? I hear several kinds of reactions. One is rage. A black woman of twenty-three said,

> Sure my periods are painful. But no doctor is gonna touch my body. They got my mother and my sister, and they're not gonna get me.

Another woman felt she had been a victim.

> It all happened so fast. I come in for a Pap test and they say "you've got fibroids and I think we should take them out," and the next thing I know, they've cut me open and my womb is gone. There's nothing I can do and I feel I'll never be the same.

The awareness of hysterectomy as a social issue can enter relationships between men and women also. One Latina woman confided,

> Sometimes I think I'd like to have a hysterectomy. I don't want any more children and my periods are terrible. But I know my husband would think I was not really a woman if I had a hysterectomy, and he would think I was a victim of the Anglo doctors.

Hysterectomy works as social control in both directions. Many of us have unnecessary hysterectomies, and for third-world women those are often prompted by racist assumptions. Yet for some of us our bad experiences with the health system make us so apprehensive that we do not seek or get care we may need.

INTERNALIZED SEXISM

The particularly frightening thing about how medicine works as social control today is the way medical and sexist ideology is internalized. No one has to come around and force people to be subservient or to act powerless, if the people do it themselves. The consciousness-raising function of the women's movement, the concept of black pride, and the attention to assertiveness are all efforts to contradict internalized sexism and racism.

Yet no one can grow up female today without internalizing sexism. We take the stereotypes of the appearance and behavior of the "ideal" woman and expect those standards of ourselves. We adopt clothing styles and standards of physical condition that keep us less powerful. We learn the rules for being "nice" instead of asserting ourselves. Many of us are moving out of these patterns of behavior, yet they are still certainly relevant for all of us.

Women internalize the sexism in the medical system also. Doctors complain that women come in seeking unnecessary treatments. Of course we do. We have been brought up to seek help from a more powerful person rather than taking charge of our own lives. Of course this carries over to medicine. Women take for granted and tolerate a much higher level of pain and discomfort than do men. It is part of female socialization to expect pain and to take personal responsibility for "psychogenic" illnesses that may in fact be organic. We "cope well" with childbirth difficulties and major surgery. It is truly useful to develop coping strategies, but one way sexism works is that women take for granted that we may experience some medical trauma during our lives. Men generally do not take that for granted. Women almost expect a hysterectomy at some point in their lives. Listen and you will hear the phrase "I had my hysterectomy. . . ."

It is not that as individuals we choose to abuse ourselves. We become part of a system in which physicians are trained to value women less and to think of surgery routinely, and where women do not challenge authority. We focus on coping with trauma rather than avoiding it. Medical ideology and sexism reinforce each other in women's experiences.

WAR ON THE WOMB

The war on the womb is a serious one and has, as do all wars, members of powerless groups as its victims. The ideology justifying this war devalues women's sexuality, knowledge, and body image. In the women's health movement we must work to stop unnecessary hysterectomies, through publicity, pressure, and education.

Chapter Five

WHAT'S a WOMAN to DO?

Jan: I feel really comfortable with my decision. I worked hard and found out all the information I could, and I asked my doctor a lot of questions. It wasn't an emergency, so I had a lot of time, and I'm sure I made the right decision.

Phyllis: I don't feel like I made the decision, although I think it was right to have the hysterectomy. I feel like my doctor decided what needed to be done and talked me into it. I think I agree, but I wish I had had more power in the decision.

Gail: I still don't know if I made the right decision. My doctor was convinced that I should have a hysterectomy, but somehow I feel like I was letting down other women by going ahead and having one. That may sound strange but it feels like I should have fought the hysterectomy in the name of all women.

Susan: So far I've made the decision not to decide. I'm wait-
            ing to see if my bleeding gets any worse and my fi-
            broids get any worse. My doctor agrees, though it's
            clear she's eager to go ahead if I decide to. In a way it
            feels like I should decide once and for all and get it
            over with, but I think I'd have a really hard time with
            that decision right now.

The decision whether to have a hysterectomy is a difficult one.
Even if the decision makes sense and you feel very comfortable
with it, it is still among the more important decisions we make
in our lives.

You deserve whatever help and support you need in making
this decision. Whatever feelings you have about the decision are
perfectly valid. If your feelings are too strong and unexpressed,
you may make decisions based on the feelings rather than your
clearest thinking. But don't censor your feelings, and don't let
yourself judge other women's feelings about the decision for or
against hysterectomy.

Among women whose thoughts about decisions are quoted
above, Jan, the first, is in a situation most women would prefer.
She feels comfortable that she did all that she needed to do to
be sure she was making the right decision, and she is glad she
did it. Jan has many opportunities unavailable to substantial
numbers of women. She lives in a large city with many women's
health resources, and she has friends who are health professionals
and could provide her information. She has had a long and
satisfactory relationship with her doctor, and her condition was
not urgent.

Phyllis, the second woman, feels as did Jan that her hysterectomy was needed and was the right thing to do, but her
relationship with her doctor was very different. Between her
doctor's manner and Phyllis's difficulty in overcoming her up-
bringing and asking many questions, she feels that she gave up
power to the doctor in making the decision. Now Phyllis needs
to express some anger about the way the decision was made, even
though she believes it was the right decision.

Gail, the third woman, finds herself taking on the struggles of all women. Her tendency in other areas of her life is to take personal responsibility for social problems. Her commitment to other women leads her to feel twinges of guilt that perhaps she has let other women down by having a hysterectomy. We must support women like Gail and reassure them that they always make the best decisions that they can in their situations.

Susan, the last woman, has taken an option concerning her decision that many of us are not told of. With the support of her doctor she has decided to wait and see. Susan knows she will be hearing many women's advice about whether she should or should not have a hysterectomy. If you know a woman like Susan, be sure to tell her you know she is going a difficult route and you support her in that.

DOCTORS AND PATIENTS

Good decision making in the doctor–patient relationship is very difficult given the nature of the relationship itself. The relationship has major power differences. It is an intimate relationship, but the intimacy is one way only. The patient is expected to reveal secret parts of her life, yet the doctor does not do the same. For most people, the doctor represents a higher social class, generally the doctor is white, and generally the doctor is male.

In making a decision about hysterectomy we should use all our resources to increase our power in the decision. But we must not forget that the situation itself works to limit the power we can feel. Do not be surprised if you leave a visit with the doctor feeling much more childlike than you normally do.

Most doctors are concerned and idealistic. They have gone into medicine because of a genuine desire to help people. However, their skills and training are actually very limited. Gynecologists are trained as surgeons, not as therapists or problem solvers or healers. Obstetricians and gynecologists feel that they must be emotionally neutral. They are trained to make decisions, not to assist in decision making. They are taught to weigh the costs and benefits of various procedures and to decide what is best for the patient. Their training causes them to approach a hysterectomy decision from the perspective of negotiating with the woman or even selling her on the hysterectomy.

Doctors are trained in an extraordinarily grueling environment. Medical students are expected to memorize immense amounts of information and are subject to routine humiliation by professors. Interns and residents are on duty for extremely long shifts, working frequently with severe sleep deprivation. It would seem unrealistic to expect compassionate, humanistic health care from people who have had often not an ounce of compassion in their training.

The system of paying the doctor will have some influence on the decision-making process. If the doctor is paid on a fee-for-service basis, for each treatment done, he or she is dependent on the patient's goodwill for more patients. Doctors may lean toward treatments that are popular but less sound medically. They are also motivated to seek a more personalized doctor–patient relationship.

In a third-party system, in which the doctor is paid a salary or in some other way is paid indirectly, the treatment can be independent of the patient's resources. This is not necessarily better for decision making. Here the doctor is more likely to behave in such a way as to please his or her colleagues and adhere to standard practices. Women who are interested in holistic health may find few doctors in traditional settings who are aware of options outside standard medical practice. To find a holistic doctor essentially means going to a doctor who is in private practice.

Diana Scully, in her study of the training of medical doctors, found that in a teaching hospital decisions about hysterectomy were influenced by the particular resident's need for additional practice. When the resident had completed the required number of cases of a particular surgery, he or she talked fewer women into it. Another strategy for obtaining cases was "saving cases," that is, keeping a particular case for the resident's own practice rather than allowing the woman to progress through the system.

Doctors are trained, consciously or unconsciously, to make decisions based on the patient's "social worth." Studies of behavior of the staff in emergency rooms show that the effort to save a person in an emergency is a function of the person's social worth. The same processes operate in the hysterectomy decision. "Social worth" is a function of factors such as the person's age and social class. Hysterectomy decisions will be influenced by the number of children the woman has and whether the doctor thinks she should be allowed to have any more children.

The list of impediments to good doctor–patient communication seems endless. Studies have shown that doctors are taught to think of women as poor reporters of symptoms and incapable of making informed decisions. In addition doctors are taught to think of themselves in a fatherly role as regards women's health care. As one doctor wrote in 1968: "If like all human beings he [the gynecologist] is made in the image of the All Mighty, and if he is kind, then his kindness and concern for his patients may provide her with a glimpse of God's image."

Part of the trend toward hysterectomy is explained by what Norma Swenson of the Boston Women's Health Book Collective calls a "club" mentality.

A woman has a group of friends her own age:
1.   One friend has a hysterectomy, done by Dr. X, who is more prominent than her own doctor.
2.   Then another friend has her uterus out suddenly.
3.   The woman feels left out, as if she is in the hands of an incompetent.
4.   She pressures her doctor or she goes to Dr. X and gets "done."

WOMEN'S DILEMMA

So what's a woman to do? The doctor says the hysterectomy is necessary or at least will help your problems. Books like this tell you to question the necessity of hysterectomy. Your doctor is very important to you, and it's important to trust him. You have for years. You have very strong feelings about your body and you do not want your body abused, yet you have real problems and perhaps a hysterectomy would relieve those problems. On the other hand, the problems aren't all that bad. Maybe you should just put up with them for a bit longer.

The dilemma is also that many of us are so tuned in to caring for other people that it is very difficult for us to care for ourselves. I hear many women wanting someone to take over and care for us in the way that we care for our children and often our husbands. The trouble is, *we* are generally the ones who are brought up to do the caring for, and we don't get it coming back to us. It is very important to try to develop strategies for dealing with this.

STRATEGIES

These are helpful basic points that women have found useful in many areas:

1. *Bring a list of questions*

For many women the main difficulty here is that we feel guilty if we take more of the doctor's time, if we don't know information we think we should know, or if our questions seem unimportant. The doctor is, after all, your employee. You have a right to expect what you need from the doctor. A written list of questions is very helpful because when you are in a stressful situation, it is hard to think. If you think ahead of time of questions that might come up and write down the answers, you will be more likely to get the information you need.

Rachel is proud of the homework she did before her doctor's visit.

> I went to the library and looked up everything I could and I talked to a friend who is a nurse. I went in with questions all written out and blanks for the answers. I wanted to know what size the fibroid was, how the doctor knew how fast it was growing, when they thought it would stop growing. It was very hard to keep asking the questions. I felt like I had a quota of three and then I should leave. But I kept it up and I'm glad I did.

2. Ask follow-up questions

Often the questions do not occur to us until after the visit. Then we want clarification of what the doctor said. Don't forget that you can call your doctor and ask questions over the telephone. Sometimes the nurse can answer the questions in a more helpful way than the doctor, but often we need to ask the doctor. Marjorie describes her strategy.

> I was very persistent. After the visit I went home and talked to a friend and made a list of questions that I wasn't able to explain to my friend. I called the doctor back the next day and he called me when he was free. I kept asking those questions and made several more calls until I was confident that I understood.

3. Bring a friend

The payoff from bringing a friend to a doctor's visit may not be very obvious. Perhaps you will have a conversation with your friend about a decision you need to make and that would be enormously helpful, but often your friend is simply there. Your friend represents a connection to your "outside self." We are able to think more clearly when there is a person we know and like who is thinking about us. And you can talk with your friend after the visit. The friend will often remember things that you don't remember, or in the discussion you will raise questions you later will have answered. Lee went with a friend as a health advocate on a doctor's visit.

> I couldn't believe how different she looked. Here was my bright intelligent friend looking totally glum and glassy-eyed and sitting there silently. I had never been an outsider in a doctor–patient interaction before. It was impressive; she was totally unlike herself. I found I added a few things to the conversation with the doctor that both of them found very helpful. And afterward I was able to remember things the doctor said that my friend hadn't heard at all.

4. Seek additional information

The women's health movement has produced a wide range of helpful information in book and pamphlet form on many topics, one of the best and long-lived of which is the Boston Women's Health Book Collective's *Our Bodies, Ourselves.* In your area there may be a women's health center or a public health clinic that has good sources of information. Even if you are using a private doctor, a telephone call to a clinic for additional information on your topic can lead you to articles, pamphlets, books, or people that could be very helpful.

5. Talk with other women

We are systematically discouraged from talking with one another. We are told that women convey misinformation; common beliefs are dismissed as "old wives' tales"; yet other women are an invaluable resource. You can tell when a woman is speaking from such bitterness that she is not thinking clearly, and you can pull out the information that is helpful to you.

Those of us who can't make those distinctions will not think very clearly about what the doctor is saying, either.

From other women we learn a broader variety of experience. Your friends will often be in the same social groups that you are in: the same class or race or age group. Their experience will have some things in common with whatever experience you would have.

Sometimes we hesitate to talk with other people because we feel that revealing ourselves will make us vulnerable to their inquisitiveness or advice. Unfortunately, that is occasionally true. We all need to be cautious that when we talk about our own experiences we do not give advice to other people. What has happened to you and the choices you have made may be far from appropriate for someone else. But do not give up on other women. As one woman said with surprise, "I told my friend about what I've been thinking about and she was very helpful. She listened to me and she had some very good things to say. I feel much less alone now."

6. *Get a second medical opinion*

This is crucial. It means finding a second doctor, making an appointment specifically for a second opinion, asking that doctor to request pertinent information from your doctor, and going for the appointment.

It is good when at all possible to obtain the second opinion from a physician in a different network from that of your regular physician. For example, if you generally see a private doctor, you can call a local clinic and find out whether they do second opinions. If they do not, they may be able to recommend a physician who would do one.

Sometimes it is useful to have a second opinion from a physician who is known for working in the area of your concern, even if that means traveling some distance, and even if that doctor is not the best doctor to do your hysterectomy. If you live near a teaching hospital, you can arrange for a second opinion from a physician who is a recent medical school graduate and up-to-date on the medical topics surrounding your problem.

Sometimes we hesitate to seek a second opinion because we think our doctor will feel offended. First of all, a doctor should not feel offended if we want additional verification, and we should not decide what is best for us based on our doctor's feelings being hurt. Second, our doctor may hint that if we seek a second opinion it is because we do not agree with his or her judgment. That may not be the case at all. It may very well be that the second opinion will confirm what the first doctor said. That was certainly true for Janet. "I chose the second doctor by asking the doctor who worked at the local women's clinic who was involved in my case who she thought was the best gynecologist in the city. The second doctor said he would have done a hysterectomy six months earlier."

Attacks on second opinion programs imply that if the second opinion recommends no surgery and the first opinion recommends surgery, women will always accept the second opinion as being the most appropriate. That also is not true. It may be that the second opinion will advise waiting and you will decide that your difficulties make hysterectomy truly urgent.

Statistics show that when people have second opinions they are less likely to have the operation than when they do not have a second opinion. That is partly because we are less likely to seek a second opinion when our hysterectomy is absolutely urgent. Second opinions often serve to assist us in deciding a difficult question. But the reason second opinions are so very crucial is that for many of us, hysterectomy may not be necessary. It may be that there are other alternatives or that we could wait and possibly not need one at all.

Second opinions are after all given by medical doctors trained to do surgery. Like the physician who gave the first opinion, they take for granted drug or surgical treatment for an illness. Nevertheless, second opinions often do convince us not to have the surgery. It may or may not be that the first doctor was a "crook." It may simply be that your situation is not clear-cut.

Even if you are fairly sure that you want or do not want a hysterectomy, I strongly recommend seeking a second opinion.

It could mean that you would not have an operation you might otherwise have had. You might end up trying another treatment or delaying surgery. It could also give you far more confidence in proceeding with surgery.

7. *Talking it through*

This strategy requires finding a person who can listen to you. It will probably be a friend. It could be a member of the clergy or a person in an official helping capacity, like a counselor. You need someone who will listen to you as you talk about your decision—someone who will not jump in at the first mention of the topic and tell you his or her experience. You need the person to sit down with you without distraction and listen to you as you think out loud. The person might ask you questions to help clarify, such as "How do you feel about that?" Or "What other information do you have?" But the listener is not there to think for you, just to assist you to think for yourself.

If you decide to use a friend in this way, I recommend specifically requesting what you need. You could say something like "I need to talk about my decision about hysterectomy. Could you please listen to me and be a sounding board. I do not want you to give me advice, but right now I want you to just listen."

8. *Advocacy*

Now let us assume that you have made your decision. You have had your hysterectomy, or you have decided not to have one. Do something with that experience! Share your thinking and your information with other women. Talk with your women friends, at the very least. You never know when something you say about your decision-making process will make an enormous difference to someone else. Be respectful of the other person and her own decision-making process, and do not assume that your decision is right for her. But too many areas and too many ideas have been kept hidden, partly because we hesitate to talk to each other.

The decision about hysterectomy is bound to be complex. Most of us struggle hard to be assertive and take charge in our lives, but here we are facing an intimately important decision in an environment that may make us feel powerless. Take whatever steps you can to take charge of your decision. Do as much or as little as you can, and push yourself a bit. And then, relax and know that you have made the best decision you can, even if you later reconsider. Make it, carry it through, and then absolve yourself of any guilt.

Chapter Six

TAKING IT OUT

You have decided to go ahead and have a hysterectomy. What will happen? What should you expect? Every woman's experience is different from every other woman's experience. Hospitals vary, doctors vary, and each woman's home and social situation will be different. Your experience may be better than the good experiences described here, or you may be very disappointed. The main thing is to be as well prepared as you can.

FEEL THE FEELINGS

Whatever the realities of your experience, you are sure to have many feelings about it. A totally routine hysterectomy, for good cause and with proper preparation, will still arouse feelings. And they may not be the feelings you expect!

You may find yourself shaking or in a cold sweat, when you know you have been reassured that everything will be all right. You may find yourself laughing hysterically for no apparent reason. You may find yourself needing to cry. Even hearing about what happens in a hysterectomy may arouse feelings for some of us, such as those Gladys expresses:

> I know I should find out about what happens in a hysterectomy, but every time I read anything I get a knot in the pit of my stomach and my hands go cold. Here I am an educated woman, fifty-three years old, and I can't face some elementary biology!

If your reaction to reading technical material is similar to Gladys's, perhaps you can find a friend who will read it over with you.

WHAT HAPPENS

Hysterectomy involves removing the uterus, or womb. Usually the cervix is removed as well.

The reason the cervix is removed is that if tissue is left inside the pelvic cavity it becomes vulnerable to infection.

Mary Ann asks a question unspoken by many women:

> I always wondered how all that stuff is taken out. What happens to the muscles and the ligaments and the blood vessels that have been connected to them? I can't imagine what my insides look like.

Mary Ann might want to figure out a way to see a nursing training film on surgery. If she makes friends with some nursing students or nursing instructors, she might get to see one if they think she can handle it.

The blood vessels are tied off, or cauterized with heat or cold, close to the closest larger blood vessel. My image is that it is like taking cuttings from a plant, when you remove the small growths and leave only the main branch. The ligaments also are cut back to the next larger portion, and the muscles are sewn back together or attached to another organ.

The upper end of the vagina is stitched together, and when the scar heals you probably will not be aware of it. The opening where the cervix was and where there will now be a scar is not at the actual end of the vagina. It is in the top portion of the vagina near the end. If you reach in with your finger and find your cervix, you will notice this.

The vagina is never removed except in extraordinary circumstances, such as invasive cancer. In some treatments for cancer it is shortened somewhat. This is called a vaginal cuff.

If the fallopian tubes and ovaries remain, they are secured with a few stitches to the top of the vagina. The ovaries continue to produce eggs, which dissipate into the pelvic cavity.

ABDOMINAL OR VAGINAL

Hysterectomy can be done abdominally or vaginally. Abdominal hysterectomy involves an incision (cut) in your abdomen. After the operation you will have a scar six to eight inches long. It may be vertical, extending from your navel down toward your pubic area, or it may be horizontal ("bikini incision") along the top of your pubic hair area.

Stephanie, who is fifty-three, talked with her doctor about which kind of incision to use.

> I told her it was real important for me to have a horizontal incision. I'm plump and I like my stomach and I didn't want it to have a line sticking out on it. My doctor said she would do it that way if she could, and sure enough she did.

An abdominal hysterectomy is chosen if the ovaries are to be removed, if there is a large tumor in the uterus, or if there is disease in the pelvic cavity. In the operation the incision opens the pelvic cavity and the flap of skin is moved aside so the internal organs can be seen and can be cut out with surgical instruments.

Vaginal hysterectomy involves propping the vagina open with instruments, positioning your body in the "lithotomy" position with your bottom up in the air and your head downward, and shining lights so that instruments can be used inside the vagina. In a vaginal hysterectomy there is an incision, but it will not be visible to you because it will be at the top of your vagina where your cervix was.

Rose had a vaginal hysterectomy when she was forty-two and had an unexpected aftermath.

> They warned me, but I still couldn't believe the backache I had after that operation! The nurse said it was because of the position I was in for the operation, but my back hurt like I thought I was going to die.

Vaginal hysterectomy is generally chosen if repairs of the vagina are necessary. Repairs may involve tightening the muscles (literally by taking a "tuck") if they have become relaxed during childbirth, or tightening the opening to the urethra if those muscles are weak and urine drips when you cough or sneeze.

The vaginal approach is especially common if your hysterectomy is because of prolapsed uterus, when the uterus descends into the vagina.

Sometimes the choice between abdominal or vaginal hysterectomy is obvious. If the hysterectomy is to correct prolapse, then vaginal hysterectomy is probably the best choice. If the ovaries are involved or the uterus is very large, then abdominal hysterectomy is the best choice.

If the choice is less clear, there are several issues to consider. Abdominal hysterectomy, because it involves a deeper anesthetic and a major abdominal incision, has a longer recovery period. Your abdominal muscles will need to recover, and that means it will be difficult for you to turn over, to push open a door, and to cough.

Vaginal hysterectomy on the other hand brings a higher rate of complications, such as damage to the urinary tract. If you look at the diagram of the pelvic cavity on page 7, you will see that the urinary tract is very close to the vagina.

It is probably true that the more experienced and skillful the surgeon, the less likely are complications from a vaginal hysterectomy. You may want to seek a second opinion about which kind of surgery is better for you. However, if your doctor strongly favors one or the other procedure, it may be that your doctor is more skillful and experienced at that kind of surgery.

IN THE HOSPITAL

Every hospitalization for hysterectomy is different. Hospitals vary from small community or religious hospitals to gigantic, highly organized bureaucratic institutions. Nursing staffs range from highly specialized teams, each nurse with a different job, to a small number of people caring for the patients. Doctors differ in their preoperative instructions, and hospitals differ in their routines.

Each woman's experience with the hospital will be different also. For some the hospital is a frightening place and the technical and scientific activity is overwhelming. For some it feels very depersonalized, and for others it is like being in a hotel. I have heard more than one woman, especially mothers who have been sick, say that staying in the hospital meant the first rest she had had for ages. Others worry about how their families are managing. Please keep all of this in mind as I outline the typical hospitalization.

You will probably be admitted to the hospital the day before surgery is scheduled. A thorough medical history will be taken, and this can be in several forms. You may have filled out a questionnaire before coming to the hospital or you may be asked to do it when you arrive. Some information may already be in a computer at the hospital, especially if you belong to a plan in which your doctor is salaried by the same hospital. You may be interviewed by a nurse or intake worker when you arrive at the hospital.

It is crucial to treat these medical-history forms very seriously. Give yourself enough time to think about the questions, and if possible take the form home ahead of time so you can fill it out in a more relaxed atmosphere. It is in the medical history that possible allergies or preexisting conditions that could be vital in your treatment will be revealed. Do not try to figure out what is relevant and what is not relevant. Give every bit of information you can think of. If you cannot take the form home, try to bring notes about significant events and dates. It is likely to be important to know when your symptoms began, when you had any other major treatment such as surgery, and when you had any pregnancies or births.

Incidentally, if you should happen to see your medical record, you may see yourself described as a "nullip" or a "multip." Those are short for nulliparous or multiparous, referring to whether you have had no pregnancies (nullip) or have had pregnancies (multip). Whether we have had pregnancies seems to be a crucial identifying aspect of women in the eyes of the health system, probably reflecting the view that woman's main function is reproduction.

Special attention in the history is paid to whether you have had allergies or lung problems. These could complicate the anesthesia.

You will also have a thorough medical examination when you enter the hospital. This may appear repetitive, since your doctor may have done one recently, but it is part of hospital procedure.

Your physical will probably include blood tests and urine tests. The blood for the blood count (CBC, for complete blood count) will probably be drawn from a vein in your arm. It includes tests of hemoglobin level (oxygen-carrying capacity of red blood cells) and a red blood cell count. In addition, your blood type will be identified so that compatible blood can be reserved for you in the blood bank. You will probably not need a transfusion, but this is one way that hospitals prepare for emergencies.

The urine test involves your cleaning your vulva and urinating into a cup. The laboratory tests the urine mainly for kidney functions. The kidneys are crucial to the body in times of stress, and the health team needs to know how well your kidneys are working.

A chest X ray is generally done on admission to the hospital. If you have had a chest X ray in the last six months or so, be sure to tell your doctor in advance, so the X ray can be used in the hospitalization. We should try to avoid unnecessary X rays at all times.

Two other tests that could be ordered are an intravenous pyelogram (IVP) or a barium enema. The IVP is a test of kidney function and the barium enema is a test of bowel function. In both tests a radio-opaque dye substance is followed by X ray as it goes through your body. The tests are unpleasant, but most women do not find them painful.

Most of these tests should be done before hospitalization. In many areas, however, insurance policies influence health care procedures, and your doctor may admit you to the hospital for these tests because that is the only way the insurance will pay for it.

Probably the night before surgery you will sign consent forms for the operation and the anesthesia. The law requires that you understand the procedure before signing consent forms. In fact, people often do not truly understand. Sometimes we need to ask for interpreters, and sometimes just plain explanations. Consent forms are generally written at a graduate-school reading level, as one expert discovered.

For some women the consent form is the worst part.

Alicia describes her experience.

> I looked at the consent form and everything went black. My English is not too good, and when I was in the hospital I could talk to the nurses because they didn't talk so complicated. But that consent form, I didn't know what it really meant or if I could not sign it.

The consent forms may include permission for any of many procedures that could be done. This leaves it up to the surgeon how much should be removed. Rachel, for example, because she had several less extensive procedures, signed a consent form for total hysterectomy several times.

> I really had to trust them. They told me they would take out only what was necessary, what was really infected, but the form I signed would have let them take everything.

Undoubtedly this kind of blanket permission is sometimes or even often used to talk women into giving permission for procedures we do not need. We may feel we want to know the results of a diagnostic procedure before a hysterectomy is done even if the surgeon thinks it is necessary. It is also true, however, that general anesthesia is very dangerous. It does not make sense to have two operations unnecessarily if we can trust the doctor to make the decisions we would want.

Some women ask to see the consent forms before going to the hospital so that they can think about what the forms say; others have a friend accompany them so they can talk it over on the spot. You may also be required to sign a consent form for sterilization. You may need to sign this several days before surgery.

This sterilization consent form represents a victory in the struggle against sterilization abuse. At one time it was common practice to talk women into sterilization when they were under pressure, and then to do the sterilization operation immediately. Hysterectomy, though not an appropriate sterilization procedure, does leave a woman unable to have children. The regulations may require consent for sterilization even though the hysterectomy is done for other reasons. Signing consent forms does *not* sign away your right to sue if you later find that you were misinformed.

The anesthesiologist is a doctor who administers and monitors the anesthesia used. Anesthesia is the process of eliminating your perception of pain so that the surgery can proceed without your body going into shock from the pain. Anesthesia is complicated and probably more dangerous than the surgery itself. The anesthesiologist will probably interview you a day or so before surgery, and will explain what is going to happen and check on problems that may affect the anesthesia. The anesthesiologist will also ask questions about your medical history.

Sometimes you may be offered a choice between a general anesthetic and a regional, usually an epidural, anesthetic. In a general anesthetic you are put to sleep; in an epidural a fluid is introduced to your spine that removes sensation from the lower half of your body. The general anesthesia puts you to sleep either by giving you a gas to inhale or by the injection of a drug into your bloodstream. An epidural anesthetic may be somewhat safer, but sometimes it is followed by severe headaches. In your process of seeking second opinions about your operation, you might discuss with other doctors which anesthetic might be best for you. The anesthesiologist also orders preoperative medication (for anxiety) for the morning of the surgery. This preoperative medication itself may cause headaches. The anesthesiologist will also ask you to sign a consent form for the anesthesia.

As Rebecca looks back on her hysterectomy experience, the visit with the anesthesiologist was the most frightening part.

> I really don't remember any problems with any other part. I had good care, and I liked the nurses and I recovered quickly, but when I was talking to the anesthesiologist all of a sudden I started getting cold sweats. I couldn't think and I didn't hear most of what he said. I had to ask the nurse later what would happen. Later that evening in visiting hours a friend came by and when I was telling her about it I found myself shaking like a leaf. It felt like I was going to die. And the anesthesiologist was the only one who could save me.

Rebecca is expressing feelings that others of us may have. However bizarre your feelings seem, let yourself feel them.

BEING A PATIENT

The first evening you will learn the hospital routine and meet the nurses who will be caring for you. In any hospital it is the nurses who provide the basic care. They are excellent sources of information about hospital procedure, medications and surgery techniques, and recuperation. Nurses, far more than doctors, are trained to educate patients. They are likely to be able to answer questions in a far more effective way than the doctors can.

You may find in asking for information or assistance from nurses that they seem to have less time for you than you would like. In nearly every hospital the nursing departments are understaffed. Fewer nurses are hired than are actually needed, and each nurse feels extremely pressed for time to do the basic work. So your request may be heard as less crucial than getting the medications out.

In addition, nurses bear the brunt of frustration patients feel toward the doctor or the hospital system. It is far easier to become irritated at a nurse than it is at a doctor. The nurses are more visible, and probably we feel less in awe of them. If you find yourself irritated with the nursing staff, try to express your irritation in a useful manner, and try to see the work pressures the nurses are under. As women workers in the health system, they do a crucial and often unappreciated job. If we as patients can be supportive to them, we will receive more information and better care.

When you are admitted, the nurse will record your vital signs—your temperature, blood pressure, pulse, and respiration. These will be recorded frequently during your hospital stay. Any valuables you may have are put into safekeeping (it is probably smart to leave them at home), and you are shown where you will be sleeping. Hospital gowns are usually available, and some women use them for daytime wear, changing to a special gown from home for visiting hours.

Ask friends who have been in the hospital about tips for making your stay more comfortable. Here are some ideas:

Bring a pillow from home! The ones in the hospital have plastic over them and are hard.

Someone bought me a fancy nightgown, but it was nylon and I was sweating so much I couldn't stand it. I had to have cotton.

My children were in preschool when I had my hysterectomy. I brought some big bright paintings they had done and some masking tape. I decorated my part of the room and it made it feel much more like home.

The nurse will ask if you need a special diet. Hospital food is unfamiliar, and many people complain. Some prefer something familiar like a Big Mac, and others find the hospital food has too much beef or starch or sugar. Many of us complain about food when we are under stress in a new environment, but in fact we can probably do quite well with the hospital diet. Do not hesitate to bring in vitamin supplements or ask your family to bring care packages of fresh fruits and vegetables during the times you can eat regular food.

If you take vitamins or any other medication regularly, be sure to tell the doctor ahead of time so he or she can write orders for you. If you take vitamin C every day, for example, the nurses will not allow you to take it unless orders have been written. Marilyn had not realized that, but dealt with the situation very assertively.

I take vitamins every day, and I knew if I stopped I would have withdrawal symptoms from the vitamin C. I hadn't realized I had to ask my doctor to write the orders, so when the nurse tried to take them away from me I said to her very firmly that I had to have the medication and she should call the doctor and get an order. It took some pushing, but she did it and the doctor ordered it.

You can refuse any treatment or medication in a hospital, even if the doctor orders it. For your own well-being you should try not to refuse when there is good reason for you to take the medication. It is, however, your legal right to refuse.

If you have been in the hospital before, you will know what preparation for the surgery involves. Being "prepped" includes a shower and then a very thorough shave of all the area to be exposed during surgery. This is to keep the area sterile. If you are scheduled for a vaginal hysterectomy, only your pubic area will be shaved. If you are scheduled for an abdominal hysterectomy, your stomach will be shaved also. You will be amazed at how thorough a shave can be!

A douche is often prescribed, and generally an enema. A douche is to rinse the vaginal area, and an enema is water introduced into your rectum to flush out any bowel-movement material there. The intestines slow down during anesthesia, and if they are full, you will be very uncomfortable after the operation. For many women the enema and the shave are the most unpleasant parts of hospital routine.

> I could take everything else. But the enema and the shave were God-awful. I'm sure my nurse was a sadist.

A mild sleeping pill is usually prescribed "on request," and the nursing staff often encourage you to take it to counteract being in a new, disturbing environment. You need not take it, or you can delay taking it until your normal bedtime. You will probably not be allowed to eat or drink after midnight.

Most surgery is scheduled for morning, and it is possible that you will be awakened very early. You will not have breakfast, and you will be given the preoperative medication. It will probably make you drowsy, and it will make your mouth dry. You will then be transferred to the preinduction room. In many hospitals you are brought in the bed that you slept in, and in other hospitals you will be transferred to another bed for the trip.

Intravenous medication (IV) is started. An IV consists of a fine needle, inserted into your wrist or arm, attached by plastic tubing to a bottle that hangs on a rack on your bed or beside you. The IV bottle may contain plain saline solution, water with the same amount of salt as in your body tissues. This is to prevent dehydration. Sometimes a sugar solution will be in the bottle, to keep your blood sugar up while you cannot eat. The anesthesia is sometimes introduced through the IV, by changing the bottle to one containing the anesthetic drug or by injecting it through a valve in the tubing. Antibiotic medications to prevent infection can also be included in the IV solution.

In the operating room you will be transferred to the operating table and will see, through your drowsy haze, the doctors and nurses who will operate on you. You will probably recognize the anesthesiologist and the surgeon, although they will probably look quite different in their surgical masks and caps.

Catherine reports:

It was weird. Here I was talking with them about my work and all of a sudden I was asleep.

You will be scrubbed well several times by the operating team, themselves having rigorously scrubbed, and the operation will begin. You will be attached to monitors, for the anesthesiologist, of your breathing, heart rate, and oxygen intake. During the surgery you will have a tube in your throat. This may cause some soreness the next day. Fewer monitors are necessary if you have an epidural anesthetic.

A hysterectomy operation usually takes about one hour. After the operation you are wheeled to the recovery room, where a special nursing team will care for you. They will record your vital signs frequently until your heart rate and breathing stabilize. Usually you wake up briefly in the recovery room and then go back to sleep immediately. When your condition has stabilized— when your vital signs are constant and you respond and are oriented—you will be returned to your room.

Usually when you get back to your room you will find you have a catheter in your urethra—a thin tube attached to a bag has been inserted in the hole from which you urinate. This is because your urinary function slows down as a result of anesthesia. The catheter allows the fluids to be eliminated from your body without your muscles needing to function properly.

For the first day or so after surgery the fluids you take in and eliminate are measured, so that any internal damage can be noticed. Jane was reminded of the times when she had had babies:

It's always a trip! You measure what you take in and then you watch that same number of cc's come out! I feel like one of those drinking and wetting dolls!

Generally the catheter is removed after the first day. Many women during the hospital stay develop urinary-tract infections from the catheter. This means additional antibiotics.

Pain medication and nausea medication will probably be ordered for every few hours if requested. The nurse is allowed to give you pain medication every four hours, for example, but gives it only if you ask for it. It is probably a good idea not to "grit your teeth and bear it." The pain medication for the first couple of days is probably very helpful to let your body heal instead of putting its energy into fighting the pain.

After the operation a number of steps are taken to prevent complications. Walking is stressed very early. This is amazingly difficult, especially after an abdominal hysterectomy with a general anesthetic. Walking is crucial, however, to stimulate breathing and circulation. The nurse will pester you to walk and may have you do exercises in the bed as well. It will feel impossible, but it is important to get moving.

You will also be told to cough. You will not believe how difficult something like coughing can be. The reason you cough is to keep your lungs clear and your breathing going. Pneumonia is not uncommon after any surgery, especially if you are a cigarette smoker. The nurse will help you by showing you how to hold a pillow over your abdomen if you have had an abdominal hysterectomy, or to cross your legs very tightly if you have had a vaginal hysterectomy. This will help reduce the pain in coughing, and you will feel less like your incision is going to burst. Trust the nurse, the incision will not burst from coughing! Additional breathing exercises are often suggested, such as blowing a fluid from one bottle to another. These exercises are to prevent atelectasis, a condition in which the lungs do not expand fully, which can lead to pneumonia.

Walking and leg-flexing exercises in the bed are to help prevent thrombophlebitis. Thrombophlebitis is blood clots that form in the legs and can travel upward and lodge in the heart or the lungs. Thrombophlebitis is especially likely among women who are older, heavy, or on hormones. It can range from uncomfortable to life-threatening.

After the operation you will not be allowed to have solid food for a few days. Your abdomen will have become sluggish during the anesthesia, and at first your only nutrition will be through the IV tube. The nursing staff will listen to your abdomen for bowel sounds. Hearing bowel sounds will assist the doctors in knowing when to allow you to have fluids and then solid foods. As your bowel becomes active again, you may experience very severe gas pains. For some women the gas pains are worse than the pain from the incision. When the gas pains hit, you tend to stiffen up, but the best thing to do is to walk or to hold onto a pillow and roll from side to side on the bed.

Ethel described a special kind of support in the room.

> It was wild! Here we were, cheering each other on, rejoicing at every fart. And normally we were such refined ladies!

Usually the IV is taken off during the second day after surgery, and you will be able to have fluids. What the hospital calls fluids is a meal consisting of juice and bouillon and Jell-O. After several days juice, bouillon, and Jell-O can get very boring. During the third or fourth days you will probably be allowed solid food. In some hospitals a couple of meals are a transition diet, with "light" solid foods, such as toast, custard, or poached eggs.

What has happened to your body? As you can tell from the precautions taken in a hospital, much of the effect on your body is from the anesthesia, but you also have a major incision through your tissue. You will have severe pain and will probably be prescribed morphine or a morphine substitute like Percodan as a pain-reliever. Your incision will be checked daily and the dressing—the bandages and medications covering it—will be changed.

The stitches may have been made with the kind of material that dissolves into your body, or it may be necessary for them to be removed several days after surgery. Extreme itching in the area of the incision is not uncommon. The incision, if you can see it, will look red and raised for some time. It usually gradually recedes, and a year or so later it is hardly noticeable.

Some people form "keloid" tissue, or scar tissue that is raised and thick. The causes of keloid are unknown, but if previous cuts or incisions have formed keloids, this incision probably will also. Black people tend to keloid more than white people.

Your responsibility for your personal care will increase every day. At first the nurses will give you a sponge bath. Progressively you will be able to do more, and more will be expected of you. You may be allowed to have a shower fairly soon, around the time the sutures and catheter are removed and you are steadier on your feet. A bath may be prohibited until the stitches heal.

A shampoo will be the most delicious feeling ever when you are able to have it. If you cannot have a shower, see if a friend will give you a shampoo in a sink. You can probably learn shampoo tricks yourself, such as using a cup to rinse your hair.

You will find that you have more attention each day for your personal well-being. At first you will hardly notice yourself, then you will have a shower and shampoo even if your hair does not turn out looking perfect. Then you will pay a little more attention to your hair and your face, and possibly get out your favorite nightgown. After a few days you may find you have the strength to get dressed during the daytime.

Patty and Michelle had opposite feelings about recovery. For Patty it was crucial to get moving quickly.

> I couldn't stand the thought of lying there looking like a frump. It was bad enough to be in the hospital, but I wanted to look normal as soon as I could. I didn't want people worrying about me and feeling sorry for me.

For Michelle the vacation from everyday routine was important.

It was so nice not to have any pressure, and I was so exhausted. The energy I had I wanted to use to be awake when my husband was visiting. I didn't care about putting on the makeup. I did what they told me to, but was in no hurry to get prettied up.

Rest in the hospital is sometimes not easy to get. The routine is unusual and the place is noisy and strange. While you are in the hospital it is probably wise to rest whenever you are not doing something else. Even as you grow stronger, plan on a rest time following even the slightest activities. After you sit up, find your hairbrush, brush your hair in bed, put the brush away, and lie back down, you will probably drop off to sleep for a few minutes. Delight in the fact that you have no obligations, and sleep and rest and think about no one but yourself. Your body needs it, and if your life is like most women's, your soul needs it too.

Immediately following surgery you may experience a number of signs of the effects of the anesthetic. These signs can resemble illness and can be frightening. They are probably normal, but do let the nurses know if you have any of them.

Nausea, hiccups, or vomiting
Shortness of breath
Palpitations or pounding heart
Tingling or numbness
Sweating or flushing
Feelings of confusion or anxiety

Visitors will be welcome and yet more exhausting than you predict. Some visitors are coming for your benefit. Enjoy a short visit with them. It is good to see someone dressed in regular clothing who talks about everyday activities at home. That's an important part of your becoming reconnected with the outside world. But let yourself fall asleep even during their visit, or as soon as you feel tired ask them to leave. It does you no good to become overtired.

Some visitors are coming primarily for their needs. They need to see that you are in fact all right. Let them chat with you about things going on outside the hospital, but be firm about the need for a short visit. In many hospitals you can have a telephone by your bed. A telephone visit can be very helpful, since visitors can reassure themselves quickly that you're all right, and it is far less exhausting for you to answer the telephone than to entertain someone in person.

Weepiness or depression in the hospital are quite common after hysterectomy. It seems similar to postpartum depression, and if you find yourself needing to cry, go ahead and cry and don't worry about what it is you may be crying about. You may be very glad to have had a hysterectomy, you may be on the road to recovery after a long illness, and yet you still may need to weep. Do not let anyone stop you.

GOING HOME

Hospitals and doctors have different routines about when you may go home after a hysterectomy. Some hospitals recommend that you go home the fifth day after an uncomplicated surgery; in others you stay until the seventh or eighth day. While in the hospital you may feel extremely vigorous, and yet just the trip home will probably be very exhausting. At home you will have a quieter environment without bright lights and a PA system, you will have more familiar food and a more comfortable bed, and you can keep your own pace. However, for many of us, at home there are children and husbands who expect to be fed, laundered, and cared for.

You will be sent home with restrictions about lifting, driving, and climbing stairs. These restrictions are inconsistent with the home responsibilities many of us have, and yet hospital staff seldom check on what arrangements we are able to make for our own care and the care of our families. Do not assume that the physician or nurse knows you have small children who need lifting, stairs between your kitchen and your bedroom, and food shopping to do. As it is likely that the main caregiver in your household is normally yourself, think very consciously about who will care for the family and who will care for you. It is before the surgery that you should make arrangements for your care when you return. Any of your friends who have been in the hospital will probably be able to offer suggestions as well as assistance. Here are some ideas:

> I cooked up a lot of food and put it in meal-size portions in the freezer. Not for when I was in the hospital—my family went out for dinner while I was away. I wanted the meals for when I got back so I wouldn't have to cook.

> I got someone to come and water my plants when I was away and got her to keep coming after I returned home.

> I made sure I was all caught up with the family accounts so I wouldn't have to worry about paying bills when I first got home.

The best recoveries from hysterectomy I have seen take place when the woman is able to have someone, like her mother or another relative, come and simply take over and care for her totally. Irene, for example, had an uncomplicated, planned hysterectomy.

> My mother came from Hawaii to take care of the house while I was away and she stayed for six weeks after my surgery. She cooked my meals and she answered the phone and she brought my mail. I don't have any children and I know I could have taken care of myself after a couple of days. But it was so reassuring to have her there.

For Pam, things were less smooth.

> It never even occurred to be that I would need special care.
> And anyway my mother and mother-in-law and sister all
> work full time thousands of miles away. My husband took
> time off work, and since he did at least half the work at
> home to begin with, he truly cared for the house and the
> children. But in our family, no one specifically cared for me.
> If I were doing it over again, I would make arrangements
> for someone else to come and care for me. And I would not
> try to feel like a hostess and make arrangements for her.

When you do go home from the hospital, you will be given a
more or less detailed timetable of activities to resume. Take the
time to go over this list and think about it carefully, so that you
can ask the nursing staff or the doctor about specifics before you
go home.

At home you will have vaginal oozing or light bleeding that
will gradually taper off. This is from the surgery site. You will be
using sanitary napkins, and although you will be sent home with
them, it is wise to get in a supply before you go to the hospital.
You may pass clots of blood or have periods of heavy bleeding.
These are probably normal, but they should be reported by
telephone to your nurse or doctor to double-check. You should
also report any fever, new pain, or odorous or excessive vaginal
discharge. All are likely signs of infection.

You will probably be given pain medication to take home, and
do not hesitate to use it as needed. However, be sure to check
on whether you should avoid any activities or substances while
taking the pain medication. It is likely that you should avoid
alcohol and drugs such as Valium or sleeping pills. You may also
experience constipation as your bowels return to normal. Try to
eat a high-fiber diet, with fresh fruits and vegetables and cereals
containing bran. You may be given a mild laxative to take home
to use if needed.

You will probably be instructed in the care of your incision.
You may be told also to avoid a tub bath for six weeks. If your

bathtub at home has no shower and the only way you can wash is in the tub, be sure to ask the nurses specifically what you should avoid if they say to avoid a bath. Douches are generally not necessary for healthy women, and should be avoided after hysterectomy in order to allow the vagina to return to normal.

You will need to learn a new technique for getting up from bed! In the hospital the bed is electric and high and does all sorts of things, but on your flat bed at home you may be surprised at how difficult getting up can be. The way to get up is to roll to one side and then use your arm muscles to lift yourself to a sitting position. Jenny discovered that technique the hard way.

> If they told me that in the hospital, I must not have been listening. There I was at home lying in my bed and the phone rang. I tried to sit up and I thought I was going to pass out from the pain. I called the doctor, and her nurse practitioner told me how to get up by rolling over.

Driving a car puts a great strain on the pelvic muscles, and in addition, driving a car safely requires very alert responses. You will probably be told not to drive a car for two weeks or more. Similarly, lifting heavy things puts a strain on the muscles that were cut in the surgery and is also a tiring activity for a body in such a state of recovery. You will be told to avoid lifting for two weeks, or four weeks. Describe your home situation to the nurse, though, because if there is no one else to lift a child into a high chair or a crib, you need to know how to carry out your daily life in the way that is safest for you.

Your own body will probably be the best guide for resuming many activities. If you have been walking, swimming, or playing tennis regularly, you will probably know when to resume those activities. They are more tiring to a recovering body. The reasons to limit them are to assist your recovery, not that doing the activity itself would be harmful.

You will probably be told to avoid "sex" for four to six weeks. It is often unclear whether you are to avoid all sexual activity or just intercourse. What about masturbation? What about sex with women? What about sex without intercourse?

Intercourse is to be avoided because bumping the stitches at the top of the vagina could be painful and bacteria might be introduced that could cause infection. Health workers seem unclear whether orgasm is harmful. Orgasm may cause bleeding, because the vagina contracts when you have an orgasm. That is probably not dangerous, although it can be frightening. Doctors need to know more about our sexuality to be able to answer questions like this appropriately.

Hot flashes are very common after hysterectomy, even if your ovaries are preserved. It is not known exactly why this happens, but it is possible that the blood supply to the ovaries is disturbed during hysterectomy.

You may find that at home you are suddenly extremely depressed or weepy. It may be that you finally feel relaxed enough to let the feelings come up. Try to reassure your family that you are fine. If you can arrange with a friend before your surgery to pay attention to you when you need to cry, you can call that friend. Remember that crying is an important healing process. It helps release feelings and relieve tensions, even if you do not know why you are crying.

Recovery times vary greatly, and one woman's experience may be quite different from another's. In one large study the average was to return to regular household activities in four to six weeks, but the time ranged up to nine weeks, especially for women over thirty-six. Unexpected severe fatigue in the first few days was common and some women found they had to stay mostly in bed for the first week. Another study showed that it was not uncommon for women to say they did not feel really back to normal for a full year, while a contrasting control group undergoing comparable operations had a much shorter recovery time.

TAKING CARE OF YOURSELF

In my counseling with women I find that most of us have not learned to take care of ourselves. We have learned to take care of other people, but we often feel guilty or uncomfortable if others offer to take care of us. We often do not even know how to ask for the care and support that we need. We feel that since we can do some things, we should not ask for assistance. Or we feel that other people's needs are greater than ours, and that once we have cared for the rest of the family, we will care for ourselves as last priority. We want to show that we are strong and healthy, and we feel this means doing things by ourselves or undertaking activities soon.

I am a great one for setting up systems ahead of time, so that no matter how we feel we will have the support we need. If we wait to arrange for assistance until after the surgery, we will probably feel that we can cope by ourselves and will not get the assistance we need.

Besides the crucial importance of rest, the specific limitations of activities, and warning signs we should pay attention to, we can take this opportunity to reevaluate our general state of health. As we all know, a healthier diet means a healthier body. Perhaps this will be the time to wean ourselves away from alcohol or cigarettes or coffee. Or perhaps we will try to substitute fresh fruit for sweet foods during our recovery. As part of our recuperation we could begin to walk a couple of blocks each day, and build that into a continuing habit.

This is your time for healing. You have been sick before your hysterectomy. The hysterectomy is a massive trauma to your system. Let yourself heal. You will probably become far healthier than you have ever been.

Chapter Seven

FEELINGS, FEARS, and GRIEF

FEEL THE FEELINGS

There is an infinite variety of feelings about hysterectomy, and they are all appropriate and acceptable. Whatever you feel is all right. In fact, whatever you feel must be expressed and acknowledged, or it may become bottled up and make problems for you in another way.

Feeling the feelings does not necessarily mean acting on them. That is a different topic, and when we are thinking about decisions, we need to act on the clearest thinking we can achieve Feelings are different. Feelings may sound "irrational." That is all right, as they are just feelings. You are not the only one who has felt similar feelings, and they do not mean that you are crazy, neurotic, or stupid.

You may feel, like Sharon, "I had a tubal ligation years ago. Why am I worried about having a hysterectomy now? I haven't been able to have children for years." You may feel, as Lydia put it, "My periods have been a big nuisance for a long time. Why am I feeling like something will be missing when I don't have them?" You may feel like Irene, "Everyone says the uterus is so important to women. I feel there must be something wrong with me because I feel nothing but delight at getting rid of it." You may feel, like Roberta, "This sounds crazy, but I'm afraid I'm going to die in the operation."

All these women are expressing normal feelings about hysterectomy. Your feelings are normal also.

Researchers have confirmed that women who are neither extraordinarily anxious nor extremely unemotional before the surgery have the fewest psychological problems afterward. That is, it is healthy to feel and express anxiety before a major operation. It is important to let yourself feel anxious ahead of time, and to have someone you can tell about those feelings who will not decide that there is something wrong with you.

When you find the person you are going to talk with, remind him or her to remind *you* that in fact you are going to be fine after the surgery and you will cope with whatever difficulties you may encounter as well as you've coped with the difficulties that you've encountered all of your life. Sometimes our fears and anxieties can be immobilizing if we forget that we do have coping strategies and have dealt with many stresses in our lives.

Rebecca is thirty-eight and has been advised to have a hysterectomy for fibroids.

> Here I was, walking around panic-stricken. My periods are terrible and I'd love to be rid of them, but I'm really frightened of doctors and knives. I did what you suggested with a friend, and when I listed all the feelings I have, it reminded me of when I had to make a decision about a job. That was a hard one too and I worried about it a lot. But I think I made the right decision. And I know I will here too.

If you are making a decision whether to have a hysterectomy or not, and you know that it is not medically critical to have one and yet it might make you feel physically better, I recommend taking a careful inventory of your feelings about hysterectomy. Spend some fair amount of time thinking about your feelings about your periods, about childbearing, about your uterus. You might make a list of the feelings in favor of hysterectomy and the feelings that might make you not want to have one. We all have very different cultural and personal experiences, and hysterectomy will mean something very different to each of us.

If you discover that most of your feelings tend toward predicting you will feel better after the hysterectomy, you probably will. If you find that as you make your list more and more concerns and worries are coming up about what the hysterectomy would mean, it might make the most sense for you to wait. No research can predict what hysterectomy will mean for you. You have all of that information, and you can retrieve a great deal of it by careful attention to what your feelings truly are.

If your hysterectomy is elective, it is crucial to evaluate your feelings as carefully as you possibly can. Hysterectomy is irrevocable. You can never change your mind. The high rate of unnecessary surgery means that many of us convince ourselves to have a major operation that is relatively optional.

Barbara did an inventory and made some discoveries.

> I hadn't thought about it that much, as my friends all seem to be having hysterectomies. But I realized I don't want to take the risks. I'm going to put it off, anyway.

Be aware that nurses and doctors are trained to encourage you to have surgery. The information they present is reassuring but based primarily on studies showing that "mentally healthy" women do not have problems. You are probably mentally healthy, yet you may have serious reactions to hysterectomy. Be sure to seek out your negative feelings as well as your positive ones.

PSYCHOLOGICAL COMPONENTS OF HYSTERECTOMY

DEPRESSION

Bearing in mind that the research is contradictory and inconclusive, one relatively consistent finding is that women tend to be more depressed after hysterectomy than after other, similar, surgery.* This depression may range from a day of weepiness in the hospital to a period of feeling low and immobilized to a severe enough reaction that professional help is crucial.

The elevated rate of depression is explained in several ways. Some people point out the great symbolic importance of the uterus to a woman's perception of herself as female. A major trauma to her female organs could cause a deep sense of loss and thus depression. Some researchers suggest that women who tend to respond to stress by becoming depressed will tend to do so after hysterectomy as well as after other kinds of stress. It may also be that there are physiological reasons, as yet unexplained, why depression may follow hysterectomy. It may be that hysterectomy can cause hormonal changes that could trigger depression in sensitive women. We need to know that there is a chance we will become depressed, so if we do have those feelings we can seek out appropriate support. It is easy for many of us to convince ourselves that any problems are due to our own inability to cope and that we do not deserve help. Surgeons also vary in recognizing women's depression. Because in many cases depression occurs significantly after the postsurgery checkup, the surgeon may not be involved at all.

* See Appendix II, "The Psychological Research on Hysterectomy."

Aline experienced depression after hysterectomy. Before her surgery she was active in the work force and very successful. She and her husband had worked in a business partnership and were reaping the fruits of their efforts. She was and remains an extremely attractive woman. When I met Aline, she was very close to tears much of the time.

> I just don't understand. I feel tired all the time and for no reason I start to cry. It seems my life has no meaning anymore. I truly did not expect this hysterectomy to affect me. I had been sterilized ten years earlier, so I knew I would not have any children, but since the hysterectomy I have just not been myself.

Two years later Aline has moved through her depression but still looks back on it.

> Yes, I am much better now. I am finally back at work and I can even smile at people now. But that was a terrible time, for over a year after my hysterectomy. I did not have a choice about the hysterectomy, but I wish I hadn't had to have it.

Aline's experience is real but far from typical. Most women do not experience major depression after hysterectomy. Yet the chance of a severe depression is a risk we must weigh in considering our own decision.

SURGERY ANXIETY

There is a large body of research information, especially in the field of nursing, that documents the feelings people have about surgery and the need for counseling. It is normal and common to feel a fear of death and to experience a crisis of confidence in the doctor. Nurses and doctors are taught to be aware of these anxieties in their patients.

Melanie describes a normal kind of presurgery anxiety.

> I had nightmares that I was tied down and cats were walking all over me. The dreams were really scary, and when I talked to a friend about them I found I was shaking. I think I might have been feeling some fears about having an operation.

BODY IMAGE

Any change in a person's body image will be experienced as stressful. When that change is as intimate as a change in reproductive organs, the stress can be considerable. If a woman has placed most of her feelings of femininity in her uterus, a hysterectomy will be more stressful than if she has placed her feelings of femininity in her breasts or other parts of her body.

I have asked women whether they would feel more disturbed

at losing their breasts or at losing their uteruses. The answers are very mixed. Freda is very sure of her response.

> What they don't see they don't have to know. I would be devastated if I lost a breast, but my uterus does not have to do with my femininity and I feel just as female now as before my hysterectomy.

Carolyn had a somewhat different response.

> It must be awful to be disfigured and to have gone through cancer like that. But I don't think I'll ever adjust to not being able to have any more children. I just don't feel right.

Whatever your experience, a hysterectomy will cause a change in body image at some subconscious level. Most of us take that in stride just as we have the changes with age or pregnancy.

Those of us who have a hysterectomy before menopause will also experience having no more menstrual periods. This is a distinct body-image change and needs some attention. Most of us are glad to have no more periods, especially if they have been painful or very heavy. But we also have many feelings that our periods are natural and that in some way it is odd not to have them. Talking with other women who have had hysterectomies can help us to express these feelings and know that we are still women and still all right. A thirty-five-year-old woman who had a hysterectomy at thirty says:

> Every now and then one of my friends will ask if I have a Tampax. It's partly a shock—"I never realized she was still concerned about that!"—but it also makes me feel like there's something secretly different about me.

CHILDLESSNESS

Sometimes people assume the only issue about hysterectomy is that a woman can no longer have a child. Women like Sally experience insensitivity in people who talk with them.

> I get so angry. People feel like they can come up to me and say, "Well, you had children, so it's all right." It makes me think the person assumes my body is for nothing other than making children. If I have made children, then anything can be done to my body and there's no problem. That's not how I see it.

Hysterectomy is about many things in addition to having children, but without a doubt, not having children is a very, very large part of what hysterectomy means. The importance for women's identity of the ability to bear children has thoroughly permeated our society. We rejoice at menstruation, because that is a sign that we are fully female and can have children. We grieve at menopause, because that is a sign that we are no longer fully functioning females, since we cannot have children. Many of us are moving away from those definitions, but no one can deny that they are very basic to our society. Women who choose not to be parents face a good deal of social criticism, even today when traditional expectations are less strong. Many women who have an unwanted first pregnancy and are considering abortion say to themselves, "Well, at least I know I can get pregnant." Freud attributed great importance to women's ability to be mothers, and although many people challenge the assumption that this is how society *should* look at women, his observations of how society *does* perceive women were extremely accurate.

The majority of research studies show that if a woman has had no children, she is more likely to feel upset after a hysterectomy than if she has had children. Yet even women who have had children often feel a sense of loss about not being able to have more. Infertility is an issue receiving increasing attention as many couples discover they are having difficulty conceiving. Infertility due to a sudden crisis is even harder to deal with. If you are facing a hysterectomy or have had one and have not had the children you wanted, I encourage you to seek out an infertility support group. There is an organization called RESOLVE, based in Boston, that offers counseling, referral, and support groups on infertility.

Another resource would be groups that help women think about adoption. You may think seriously about adopting a child after a hysterectomy.

The positive side of infertility is that for the first time in many years a woman need not be concerned with contraception. For many women contraception has been either a nuisance, if she has used a barrier method, or a worry, if she has used the pill or an IUD. Even here, though, one woman in a research study was very fastidious and upset because now that her husband did not need to use condoms anymore, she got the "dirty deal."

Women have feelings about childlessness whether or not they have had children. Ruth, for example, is forty and has had three children.

> Maybe it is because the children were so important to me, but even though I know menopause was close I just can't get adjusted to not being able to have children. It doesn't make any sense, but I feel less useful.

Pam was twenty-two when she was diagnosed as having cancer, and she has had no children.

> Well, it certainly changes your life! I feel that I am adjusting just fine, and it means I won't have to think about the choice, but I do wish that I had the option.

Donna had one child.

It doesn't seem fair. I had a beautiful pregnancy and I was looking forward to two more. Why does it have to be me who has to think about adoption? I know so many women who hated their pregnancies and hated giving birth. It's just not fair.

Lynn is furious.

Here I was, faithfully using an IUD so I could put off having children until my husband and I were ready. Then I get an infection and it leads to a hysterectomy. I am so furious, I'm beside myself.

Hazel is at the other end of the spectrum.

I had worried and worried about contraception. I had been using a diaphragm and foam since my children were born, but I know it was going to be a long time until menopause. I was thinking about sterilization when this hysterectomy came up. I think it is a blessing in disguise. Now I don't have to worry about having any more children.

Your experience, and the experience of women you know, may be similar to the voices here or it may be very different. Be sure as you listen to women speak that you let them know that their experience with childlessness is true and important.

MEN'S REACTIONS

How do men react to hysterectomy? Very little has been written, but what is mentioned is that some men have very strong reactions. Several studies discuss women whose mates leave them after their hysterectomies, taunt them with being "half a woman" or "neutered," or refuse to have intercourse with them. The concern about the reaction of men to this surgery has led some women in my studies to lie to their husbands about hysterectomy. Becky, a thirty-five-year-old woman, says,

> I'm going to visit my sister for a month. He's never going to know I'm having a hysterectomy. From what he said about other women, I know he'd disappear in a flash.

Lisa told her husband she was having a hysterectomy but not an ovariectomy.

> If he knew my ovaries were gone, I think he'd think I was no good in bed anymore.

Michelle is thirty-six, and her hysterectomy was done when she was thirty. She says,

> Well, now my husband wants a divorce, and he says the hysterectomy cost him a marriage. I feel like it's probably right for us to get a divorce, but I do feel bad. He told me a couple of times that he would never get over my hysterectomy.

Most men are very concerned about the women they love, but they have questions that often remain unanswered.

Ed was shaken by his wife's hysterectomy.

> It really upset me to see her in the hospital. All of a sudden she looked like she was almost dead. She was dopey, she couldn't move, it was very upsetting. I felt scared when she came home that I wouldn't know how to take care of her and that she was so weak. She's back to normal now, thank God!

Fernando was concerned about injuring his wife after the surgery.

> They talked to her in the hospital, but no one talked to me until I met the woman at the clinic. She told me that after six weeks we could have sex and it wouldn't hurt her. I was very afraid that I would break her open or hurt her somehow. I still feel like I have to be extra gentle.

Bob and the woman he lives with took on the hysterectomy as a joint project.

> I went with her to visit the doctor and was there right after the operation was over. I tried to find out all I could about how to take care of her afterward. It was probably helpful for her, but mostly it helped me to be involved and not feel so powerless on the sidelines.

Howard has left his wife since the hysterectomy.

> I can't tell how much was the hysterectomy and how much we just grew apart, but she just didn't seem as sexy as she had been. I tried, but I just couldn't do it. Sex was painful for her, which is a real turnoff.

Childlessness is an issue for men as well as for women. Ralph was living with a woman when she had a hysterectomy for cancer.

It's ten years ago now and I've grown a lot. When I realized Cathy would never have my child, it was a terrible blow. I feel guilty for leaving, but how could I have given her what she needs when I really wanted a child?

Richard's wife recently had a hysterectomy at thirty-five for fibroids.

I don't talk about it to anyone. None of my friends knows she had a hysterectomy. I feel ashamed, like I am less of a man or something. And we have three beautiful children and had no plans for more. I don't understand.

More research on men's feelings about hysterectomy must be done. It might very well show that most men do have significant feelings about hysterectomy itself and its effect on the women they love. One of its results may be to explain further the reactions that women have. It is often assumed, without considering the man's actions, that any problems a woman has are because of her own lack of adjustment. Furthermore, men whose partners are undergoing hysterectomy need support themselves.

GRIEF AND GRIEVING

"But I won't have any of those problems. I'm well adjusted, not too attached to my uterus, well informed, and the people around me are supportive. I won't have any of those psychological problems after hysterectomy." But you may. And whatever experience you have after hysterectomy, you deserve support in dealing with it.

Women report two kinds of experiences with depression after hysterectomy. One is a weepy day in the hospital soon after the operation. I have not seen any studies with a clear explanation for this weepiness, but many women experience it as similar to postpartum depression.

If you find yourself needing to cry in the hospital, it may be difficult to find someone who will let you. Many women feel they are a bother to the nurses, who are already rushed. It may help if before the surgery you arrange with someone and tell him or her that you may need to cry after the operation and that they should simply pay attention to you and not get worried about it.

What if you find that it's three months after your hysterectomy and you still don't feel back to normal? You are more tired than you think you should be, you need to cry often, you have very little energy and absolutely no interest in sex. You went for your six-week checkup, and your gynecologist pronounced you fine and ready to go back to work. But everything seems an enormous struggle. Your sleep is disturbed when you suddenly feel very hot.

If you do find yourself in this situation, be sure to read Chapter 9 on home-brew estrogen. It may be that your estrogen supply was disrupted, even if your ovaries were not removed. My suggestions for caring for yourself may help to relieve difficulties you may be having.

Reasons for hormonal turmoil after hysterectomy are not clear. Some researchers think that even in the removal of only the uterus, not the ovaries, the blood supply to the ovaries is disturbed. Another theory is that the uterus itself does produce hormones. In either explanation your body is adjusting to a far more drastic change than if you had had your appendix out.

Often if our bodies are telling us to rest, we experience it as depression because we do not have the energy for our normal activities. If it is any help, you should know that many women have gone through experiences like yours, and after six months to a year, they do feel far better.

This is another situation in which a support group could be extremely helpful. Some of your friends may have bounced right back after a hysterectomy and had no lingering difficulties. A support group of women who have had hysterectomies would let you hear a broader variety of experiences.

What about severe depression? A woman who is severely depressed may not even pick up this book, because she may not associate the depression with her hysterectomy. Only a very small proportion of women, possibly 5 percent, become severely depressed after hysterectomy. Many of them do not associate their emotional stress with the hysterectomy, because the hysterectomy was some time in the past. If you or someone you know is feeling a great deal of stress and did have a hysterectomy, it might make sense to proceed as if part of her difficulties were in some way related to the hysterectomy.

How do you recognize depression? If you or someone you know has had a hysterectomy and you are wondering if you may have a definable depression, how do you judge? Some of the indicators of depression are sleeping much more or less than usual, eating much more or less than usual, and periods of unexplained great sadness.

Depression is unlikely to be recognized by a gynecologist, but a counselor or psychiatrist may be able to offer some support. There are antidepressive drugs such as Elavil, which relieve some symptoms. Drugs such as Valium and Librium are tranquilizers. They may relieve anxiety, but they do not relieve depression. Valium and Librium are the most highly prescribed drugs in the world, and most of the prescriptions are written for women patients. They might be helpful when used very selectively, but the very large number of us who become essentially dependent on those drugs shows many doctors prescribing a minor tranquilizer rather than assisting us more effectively. Many women today, however, are seeking to restore their emotional balance by methods other than drugs. If you search, you will find suggestions that may help you to heal your emotional state without the use of dangerous drugs.

RAGE

It may be more socially acceptable to feel depression than to feel rage, and yet many or most of us who have hysterectomies experience feelings of rage. We feel angry because this happened to us. We may feel angry at the doctor for not taking better care of us. We may be enraged at whatever it was that caused our hysterectomy, especially if it was an avoidable event. Perhaps we know or suspect that our hysterectomy may have been unnecessary. Perhaps infertility is a very special grief for us. In each of these situations we can expect to feel enormous surges of rage.

For many women depression or sadness and sluggishness may well be rage turned inward. It may be, when we are feeling sad or sorry for ourselves or self-critical, that if we had permission we would express enormous rage. We may feel rage at a particular person or a particular event, or we may feel a generalized rage.

It is important to be able to express the fury we feel. Expressing anger is frequently not easy for women. We have been socialized to be self-critical or depressed instead of feeling or expressing anger.

Sometimes when we get close to feeling anger we feel a surge of enormous fear. The fear probably comes from times when we were very young and did express anger and something terrifying happened to us. So today the hint of rage brings up those old terrified feelings, and we choose a different way of expressing our feelings, one that worked for us as a survival mechanism when we were little.

We may feel furious with someone close to us when our rage is actually far more generalized. I would like to see us all in situations in which we could express the rage we feel without hurting someone else's feelings. But since most of us do not have that situation, it is probably better for us to express the anger we feel, even if it may be misplaced. Our husbands or children will survive our "grouchiness," and we will get the feelings out.

Some women have close friends to whom they can say, "I need to unload a little" and proceed to rant and rave. This takes the lid off the steam bubbling up inside us, so we can think more clearly about what we actually need to do.

It may be that we need to take an action because of what has happened. It is to be hoped that we can take that action in the most effective way, which may even include screaming at the person we're angry at. Because of our socialization as women it probably makes sense for us to use the rule "When in doubt, express anger." We may sometimes express our anger inappropriately, but we are far more likely not to express it at all.

Even if your hysterectomy was necessary and healing and you had a good experience in the hospital and good recovery, anticipate the need to express rage about it.

GRIEF WORK

You may not have feelings of depression after a hysterectomy. You may not feel much anger. But you still need to grieve. A person needs to go through a grieving process upon losing any body part. This process is similar to that after the death of a loved one. You will probably go through some of the same stages as in other grief work. You may not want to believe that it has really happened. You may have times when you need to cry a great deal. You may feel furious at the uterus for being defective, as you might feel furious at a person for dying.

How do you facilitate grieving for yourself or someone you

care about? One of the main ways is to give yourself permission. All the feelings that you need to feel, crazy though they may seem, are important and necessary to express.

If at all possible, set up situations where it is all right to express those feelings. Here is where a support group can be very valuable. You may be able to talk or cry or rage about your experiences in a situation where there is more safety because other women have had similar experiences.

You may also find a one-to-one situation valuable. You may be able to exchange attention with a friend. You could set aside a specific time when you listen to her and what she needs to talk about or cry about in her life, and then you trade places and she listens to you. If you find yourself the listener in a situation like this, keep an eye out for the signs that there are more feelings to express, such as the beginnings of tears, trembling lips, agitated talking, and so on. If you notice that, let the person know it's all right to express the feelings. You can hold out your arms for a hug and say, "Do you need to cry?" Or you can say, "Here, beat on this pillow, it'll make you feel better."

There is still a stigma involved in seeking professional counseling. We often feel that if we were really together we wouldn't need it, or that seeking a counselor shows there is something wrong with us. But professional counseling for a short time after any kind of grief experience can be extremely helpful. You might check with the local women's center to see whether there are specific groups for women in transition or women coping with losses. If you seek an individual therapist, interview the person carefully. Make it clear to the counselor that you are interested in short-term counseling specifically to clear away any feelings that remain about your hysterectomy.

You may be interested in being part of a support group, but cannot find one. Start your own! The main thing to remember in any support group is that no one, even the facilitator, should comment on what a woman is expressing. If a woman is expressing her feelings, those are her feelings. Even expressing sympathy can be the wrong thing to do for a woman who feels very independent and simply needs to talk.

Fears and feelings are part of every woman's hysterectomy experience. You will probably not have major problems, but you might. The best way to prevent posthysterectomy problems is to avoid unnecessary surgery. Whatever problems you do experience, you deserve help in dealing with them.

Chapter Eight

SEXUALITY!

I have three things to say about sexuality after hysterectomy or castration. One, there are changes. Two, the changes may or may not cause problems. Three, we can surmount the problems we may have, and we deserve the help we need in doing it.

But what are we told about the effect of hysterectomy on our sexual feelings? Here are some statements written for the public by medical professionals.

> Sexual gratification . . . is in no way affected by the surgical removal of the uterus.

> •

> The majority of women should have the same sexual reactions after the uterus is removed (and/or the ovaries) as before surgery.

> •

A woman—especially if she is in her twenties or thirties—can expect to be as sexually responsive as she was before she developed her symptoms.

•

Sex should not feel any different to you or your partner as a result of surgery.

•

Apart from mental and emotional variables that can adversely affect sexuality, there is no scientific basis to support the idea that the removal of the uterus has an effect on sexual response.

The message is very clear: Hysterectomy has no effect on our sexual functioning. That is the message repeated in nearly every article and book for the general public. Some writers, generally feminists and those more aware of women's sexuality, are more cautious.

For women whose uteruses have an active role in their sexual response, a hysterectomy may affect sexual sensations.

•

There is no relationship between enjoyment of sexual intercourse and the presence of reproductive organs. Sexual desire and desirability do not disappear.

Even in these statements, which I believe are accurate, it is easy to assume the writer is saying there will be no change in our sexuality.

Some of the writers want to reassure women that our sexual functioning will not be destroyed after hysterectomy. Some of the writers are simply ignorant about female sexuality and the effects that removing the uterus might have. And some writers and some doctors are probably just plain unconcerned about the effects of hysterectomy on a woman's sexuality.

Recent research documents that 33 to 46 percent of women who have hysterectomies are adversely affected sexually because of physical changes from the hysterectomy. There are two primary reasons for this. For some women, removing the internal structures creates a sense of loss. Second, for some women the loss of hormones from the ovaries, especially androgen, causes a reduction in libido.

FEMALE SEXUAL RESPONSE

Current physiological researchers describe four phases in the human sexual response cycle. The male and female response cycles parallel each other. The physical changes caused by hysterectomy may or may not be noticeable to you. Removal of the ovaries as well will cause additional changes in the response cycle. And some women who have retained one or both ovaries experience physical changes similar to those that would take place if their ovaries had been removed.

The stages of female sexual arousal identified by sex researchers William Masters and Virginia Johnson include excitement, plateau, orgasm, and resolution. The uterus is involved in each of these stages. During the excitement phase, blood rushes into the entire pelvic area. This process is called vasocongestion, and it causes the feeling of arousal. It is more visible in a man, since it causes the erection of the penis.

Women are aware of the role of the uterus in vasocongestion at times when the uterus is in a special state. Some pregnant women experience heightened sexual excitement, possibly because there is additional tissue in the pelvic area to become engorged with blood during the excitement phase. Also, women who have pelvic infections and internal scar tissue report sometimes that they are more intensely excited sexually than before their illness, again possibly because there is additional tissue that becomes engorged during excitement.

Jeanne, who had a pelvic infection and then a hysterectomy at twenty-eight, put it this way:

> It was really weird now that I think back on it. Before my hysterectomy I was turned on a lot, but orgasm hurt like hell. I just felt like I kept reaching for relief, that somehow there was a hurt inside me that orgasm would help. Sort of like an itch that you know will hurt when you scratch it but you have to scratch it anyway.

After hysterectomy, when the uterus is not there, less tissue becomes engorged with blood. There may be less sensation of arousal due to reduced vascocongestion. Jeanne noticed the change.

> Since the hysterectomy I just feel less full and heavy inside. I just don't feel as turned on. In a way it was worse before, because orgasm hurt. But now I feel like my excitement is just in the outside parts of my body, not inside anymore.

During the excitement phase the uterus is elevated in the pelvic cavity. The inner portion of the vagina balloons, increasing in diameter by as much as three times, and in length by as much as an inch. After hysterectomy there is no elevation of the uterus, and the scar tissue replacing the cervix is inelastic, which may prevent the full ballooning of the vagina. After a hysterectomy the vagina may be shorter. For some women who have had radical surgery for cancer, the vagina is quite shortened, further limiting expansion.

You should realize that the vagina can accommodate a penis even if it has not increased greatly in size. Frequently we think that our vagina is a tube open at all times, as is generally indicated in diagrams about menstrual tampons. In fact, the folds of the vagina are soft. If you put your finger into your vagina, you'll feel it around all the sides. If you put two fingers or three fingers into your vagina, it will accommodate them also. If after hysterectomy your vagina does not "balloon" as much as before your hysterectomy, it can still accommodate a penis or fingers. The ballooning may affect your sexual feelings, but it should have no effect on what you do with your vagina.

The third characteristic of the excitement phase for women is an increase in vaginal lubrication. This lubrication does not come from the uterus, and it does not come from a man's secretions. It "sweats" out of the walls of the vagina. Lubrication for a woman is the first sign of sexual arousal. It is parallel to erection in a man, as that is the first sign of a man's sexual arousal.

Vaginal lubrication is hormone-related. If you are past the menopause, or if your ovaries have been removed, the lubrication is slower to appear and less copious. For many women this change is not noticeable because so many other things are so much better after hysterectomy or menopause. But there is a physical change, and research documents that vaginal lubrication is related to estrogen level.

This is obviously relevant to you if you are having your ovaries removed. If you have a simple hysterectomy, you may not notice a change in lubrication. I mention it, though, because some premenopausal women who have had hysterectomies do notice that lubrication is less plentiful or slower to start. Similarly, some women experience hot flashes even though they still have their ovaries. Recent research shows that simple removal of the uterus has a hormonal effect.

Muscle tension in the pelvic area is heightened during excitement and plateau also, and women notice strong contractions of the muscles in the outer part of the vagina, the buttocks, and sometimes the abdomen. The "orgasmic platform" is the term for the process of engorgement and swelling of the tissues surrounding the outer third of the vagina. The outer part of the vagina prepares to grip a penis tightly, while the inner part of the vagina opens and "balloons."

The next stage of female sexual response is the plateau phase. During the plateau phase the uterus becomes elevated farther in the pelvic cavity and the inner part of the vagina balloons more. The uterus expands, becoming as much as twice its normal size. This extra increment of sexual tension will not be felt by a woman after hysterectomy. You may, of course, never have been aware of your uterus elevating in your pelvic cavity or your vagina ballooning. After hysterectomy you may realize that something is different, or you may never notice any change at all.

Women have varying responses to this information. It is not easy to talk about sex, and for many of us it is very important to remain cheerful after surgery. Yet often if one person breaks the ice, others find it helpful. Nancy, who is forty-eight said,

> I'm really uncomfortable dissecting sex that way. For me sex is better since my hysterectomy, and I really don't like to think about all the different parts. It makes me feel like I'm in a laboratory.

Christine, who is forty-one, responded,

> Yes, I know what you're saying, Nancy, but what Susanne just said helped me a lot. I've noticed that things seem different, but I haven't been able to put my finger on it. It just feels like there's less going on in there than there used to be. I remember the buildup and how all my attention would go to my middle. Now my attention is much more on just reaching orgasm. The buildup is much less strong.

The peak of sexual excitement is the orgasm phase. During orgasm women experience rhythmic contractions of the engorged tissue around the outer part of the vagina. The uterus also contracts rhythmically.

Sex researchers have found that the more severe the contractions of the uterus are and the longer the contractions continue before tapering off, the more intense a woman perceives an orgasm to be. This suggests that after hysterectomy, orgasms may not reach the intensity that they had before. The uterus is a very strong muscle, and the absence of its contractions might be noticeable. Also, if the intensity of the uterine contractions is related to the perceived intensity of the orgasm, then even if the uterus's absence is not noticed, the woman may feel the orgasm to be less intense.

Women have been aware for centuries of the fact that the uterus contracts with orgasm. Masturbation or lovemaking to orgasm has long been suggested as a technique to relieve menstrual cramps. Orgasms during pregnancy have a unique character because of the increased size of and blood supply to the uterus. It is logical to assume that removing the uterus would also affect orgasm.

Women who have experienced premature menopause talk with me most frequently about changes in orgasm. One woman who was twenty-eight when she had a hysterectomy and ovariectomy said,

> I felt very turned on in the hospital and I masturbated, but when the orgasm came it felt very superficial. My sex life is pretty good now, but the orgasm still isn't the same.

A woman who had a hysterectomy because she had had pain with orgasm for many years says,

> The major benefits? No more pain with orgasm. No more cramps. Sexuality? Orgasms aren't very strong. It is hard to achieve multiple orgasms now.

Edna, who is forty-eight and who had a hysterectomy for fibroids, says,

> I know some women have lots of orgasms but I never did. My orgasm, though, was the best thing. It was slow and deep and brought this tremendous feeling of relaxation. I would feel like all the tensions in me were melting away. Now it just doesn't have that power. It sounds disloyal, but it even affects how I feel about my husband. When I would have an orgasm I would feel this outpouring of love

for him. And now, I really do love him just as much, but that outpouring feeling just isn't there.

Gayle was fifty-one at the time of her hysterectomy for fibroids. About her sexual responses she says,

> There is less urgency. Before my hysterectomy I had two types of orgasms—clitoral and cervical—but afterward my orgasms were mainly clitoral. I'm not saying a clitoral orgasm isn't nice, because it is . . . but I just miss the combination of the two. Oh, I might add that lovemaking was painful at first. The pain was similar to belly cramps. I suppose, though, it could be a result of the bladder infection that I had. Before the operation I had a lot of pain while having sex. Now the pain has gotten better. I have less vaginal lubrication, and I use hormone cream. It comes in handy when I feel it's necessary. All in all, I think sex is less satisfying since my hysterectomy. I don't enjoy sex in as many different positions as before my hysterectomy. My vaginal canal is more shallow and that doesn't help either. Sometimes—when we really get into it—I feel as if there is something tearing or pulling. Before the operation I didn't experience this. Having sex has been better in that there has been less pain. I can feel free now . . . not so uptight with the anticipation of some sort of pain. It has been less good in that I miss having the two orgasms I told you about. All in all, I guess I'd say it's been better in some ways and worse in others.

Gayle speaks of an important distinction that few writers have acknowledged. Many women experience two kinds of orgasms: those primarily from clitoral stimulation and those from pressure on the cervix and movements of the uterus. For women whose orgasms are more internal, hysterectomy, even without ovariectomy, will have a severe effect.

Information on the two kinds of orgasms has been hidden, partly because of the rage women felt at the assertion by psychoanalyst Sigmund Freud and others that clitoral orgasms were "immature" and that the mature orgasms were vaginal orgasms. Sex researchers had documented the fact that the inner part of the vagina has no sensation, and women were angry when they were told that the kind of orgasm that can be achieved by masturbation is immature and women's sexuality depends on men. Now we are more able to separate the biases from the accurate information. *The Hite Report,* Barbara Seaman in *Free and Female,* and Singer's *The Goals of Human Sexuality* point out the fact that many women do experience internal orgasms.

These orgasms are triggered by rhythmic pressure by a penis, a finger, or some other hard object. This causes movements of the uterus and its supporting ligaments, which in turn stimulates the peritoneal membrane that surrounds the uterus. The peritoneal membrane is thought to have great pleasurable sensitivity.

Although no researchers as yet have determined the proportion of women for whom the internal orgasms are primary, for those women hysterectomy brings significant losses. There may be a relationship to the proportion of women (about 40 percent) who report decreased sexual response after hysterectomy.

Men also sometimes perceive changes in the sexual response of the women they love. A young man interviewed on the subject said that he thought his fiancée's sexual response after the operation had become more "diffused and spread out." He said that his fiancée used to have more "well delineated and focused" orgasms.

Eddy's wife had a hysterectomy when she was fifty-three. When asked whether surgery affected their sex life, Eddy says,

> No. Not at all. Our sex life has always been good. Although in some positions it was painful for her . . . but that didn't stop us one bit. We just worked around it. Sex was always good—before and after her hysterectomy. . . . We couldn't wait until we could have sex again! It was just as it always had been . . . great! The pain never presented any real problems to notice any change . . . about the only thing that was different was the new spontaneity that came from not hav-

ing to worry about any birth control. Emily had been using a diaphragm. And that makes things a lot nicer . . . a lot freer.

Of course, these quotes are from people who feel comfortable talking about the specifics of their sexual responses and who have noticed changes. Many women do not notice these changes. For example, Irene, who is forty-four, says,

If you look for trouble, you'll find it. I think my sex life is just as good as before, and I don't notice any changes.

The final stage of sexual response for men and women is the resolution phase. Here the sexual tension and engorgement of blood gradually recede. In women additional orgasms can follow the first orgasm, especially if they maintain plateau-level sexual tension. After hysterectomy, since there is less vasocongestion than with an intact uterus, it may be that the sexual tension recedes more quickly. It could be predicted that multiple orgasms would be less likely after hysterectomy than before. Some women do describe that change.

After considering the female sexual response and the role that the uterus plays in each stage, it was apparent to me that writers and doctors who say to us that there will be no change must be speaking from ignorance or bias. And yet many writers, and even more doctors, continue to report that there will be no change. For instance, Lucienne Lanson, an obstetrician and gynecologist, says in her book *From Woman to Woman: A Gynecologist Answers Questions About You and Your Body*:

Does removal of the uterus lessen a woman's ability to enjoy sex?

There is no denying that a few women do attribute their lack of sexual interest or ability to be aroused to their hysterectomy. These women almost without exception have a history of some sexual maladjustment, often the result of pre-existing psychological factors. Apart from mental and emotional variables that can adversely affect sexuality, there is no scientific basis to support the idea that the removal of the uterus has an affect on sexual response.

. . . In fact, women who have had a hysterectomy still report feeling pleasurable *uterine* contractions along with the vaginal contractions and other pelvic throbbing at the time of orgasm. The explanation for this interesting phenomenon, although not completely understood, may be the result of a conditioned response. In other words, if a woman was previously aware of uterine contractions during orgasm, the same physical sensation may occur even in the absence of the uterus.

Passages such as this, repeated many times by doctors in practice and in print, are extremely frustrating to me. Some of the points are true. But the first part clearly implies that if a woman notices sexual changes, it is her fault. For one thing, if a woman does have a strong attachment to her uterus and feels she cannot be sexually excited without it, she needs support and not to be blamed as being sexually maladjusted. And second, I don't see how anyone can say the removal of the uterus has no effect on sexual response. It may, as I keep insisting, not cause problems. But it does have an effect.

I certainly have not met any women who feel uterine contractions after hysterectomy despite Lanson's assertion to that effect. In fact, a psychologist with a different orientation from Lanson might well analyze such statements as indicating that the woman was experiencing a neurotic "phantom uterus" or even as a sign of hysteria.

We must make our doctors, including Lanson, more accountable for the misinformation they print. I put greater emphasis on possible negative changes because I do not see them talked about anywhere, and because I have met so many women who are trying very hard to figure out what they did wrong to cause the physical changes that they noticed. I fear that ignoring possible negative changes does far more harm than acknowledging them and giving ideas about how to deal with them.

COMPLICATIONS

In addition to the changes, noticed or unnoticed, that occur when the uterus is removed, a woman may be unfortunate enough to experience complications of the surgery itself. The rate of complications following hysterectomy is very high, estimated by different researchers at anywhere from 20 to 45 percent. These rates include the small proportion of women who die from hysterectomy, estimated at 0.1 to 0.5 percent.

Of the other complications, some may have a direct or indirect effect on a woman's sexual experience. Wound infection, though normally cured fairly quickly, can delay resumption of sexual activity. Urinary complications are quite frequent after hysterectomy, especially after vaginal hysterectomy. These can include injury to the bladder or to the urethra, through which urine passes out of the body. If you happen to sustain an injury to your urinary organs, the vasocongestion or extra blood of sexual arousal or pressure of penetration by a penis can be uncomfortable or painful. Similarly, if after the surgery you have difficulty urinating, your bladder can be painful during sexual activity. Other documented complications include joint pains and bone and muscle changes.

Masters and Johnson have pointed out an even more direct effect on sexuality after some hysterectomy procedures. If the surgeon in repairing the vagina does not position the vaginal cuff (or the stitches) in the upper wall of the vagina, where the cervix was, a penis can strike the scarred area, which cannot balloon in a normal way, resulting in considerable pain. Masters and Johnson describe seeing this incorrect surgical procedure among many women who report painful intercourse after hysterectomy.

CASTRATION

If both your ovaries are removed (ovariectomy, oophorectomy, or surgical castration), immediate menopause occurs and certain sexual changes that even the doctors writing for the lay public mention do take place. Some women notice these changes even if one or both ovaries are retained.

Estrogen replacement therapy (ERT), using drugs such as Premarin, is generally prescribed to counteract some of the effects of removing the ovaries in a premenopausal woman. Androgen therapy is also sometimes used. Hormone replacement therapy is very controversial, however, because of its possible links with cancer, and some women prefer to limit or avoid its use. I discuss this more in the next chapter on home-brew estrogen. Women with a history of hormone-related cancer cannot take estrogen at all.

The most noticeable sexual effect of reduced estrogen level is that vaginal lubrication is reduced and takes longer to appear. This is significant, because lubrication is the first indication of sexual tension for women. Slower lubrication not only can delay the accommodation of a penis without pain but can also make sexual stroking of the vulva painful. Slower lubrication can be a problem for any woman, but when it changes very suddenly it is particularly hard to deal with. We all develop sexual habits, especially if we are with one partner, but even by ourselves or with other partners we have certain expectations of ourselves. When a physical response changes suddenly, it is very easy to look for psychological causes or blame ourselves. Couples find they need to relearn "foreplay," and some women who had masturbated regularly say that after ovariectomy it takes so much longer to reach orgasm that they become very discouraged.

Janet had her ovaries and uterus removed when she was twenty-five. She says,

> I masturbate because I know I should, but I've taken to reading while I do. It takes so long for me to come that I get really bored compared to before.

Natalie, thirty at the time of her ovariectomy and hysterectomy two years ago, is in the same marriage that she was in at that time.

> My husband and I never thought about getting me turned on. I was always wet, and sometimes would even have an orgasm by the time he came inside me. Now there are times when I don't have any orgasms at all, and he isn't very good at getting me turned on. And then I get embarrassed and nervous and it escalates. We'd probably be fine if we started over now, because I know from my women friends that I still get aroused as quickly as some of them, but both of us have the habits from before.

Ngosi is thirty. She spoke up in one discussion.

> I'd like to put a word in here. I didn't have a hysterectomy, but I am diabetic and get a lot of vaginal infections. When I get an infection, I don't lubricate very well at all. I am a lesbian, so I'm not talking about lubrication for intercourse but lubrication for me being turned on. What I find is that when I'm not lubricated the performance anxiety comes up and I get very self-critical and worried about my sexuality.

With low estrogen level the vaginal walls become thin rather than thick and corrugated. This change along with the reduced lubrication can make intercourse painful. The thinner walls of the vagina can also lead to bladder irritation following intercourse. Even if you take estrogen, it is possible for your bladder to be irritated after penetration if you are not sufficiently aroused beforehand.

There is generally less vasocongestion during the excitement and plateau phases of a postmenopausal woman's sexual cycle, even if her ovaries and uterus both are intact. Similarly, orgasm in postmenopausal women often includes fewer contractions. Both of these can contribute to a feeling of reduced arousal.

The vulva includes the whole fleshy area around your crotch. The fatty pad around the vulva thins out as the estrogen level drops. This affects the general level of arousal, as there is less vasocongestion in the area around the vulva. In postmenopausal women the labia, or outer lips of the vagina, become less swollen during intercourse.

One function of the swelling of the labia is to transmit the rhythmic movements of the penis in the vagina to the clitoris, a very important part of satisfaction during intercourse.

After menopause the labia generally are less fleshy than before. (Some women find that jeans fit more loosely than before menopause!) In addition there is less increase in congestion in those areas during sexual arousal. Both of these changes may be noticeable, especially to a woman who has had orgasms during intercourse previously.

When the labia become thinner, sometimes the clitoris is left more exposed. Some postmenopausal women find that stroking the clitoris is very painful because it is no longer protected by the labia.

Sharon has an unusual method for solving her lubrication difficulties since hysterectomy and ovariectomy.

> Now that I have a woman lover, we share her lubrication and it's not painful to be stroked anymore. But sometimes I feel very jealous of her juiciness.

The ovaries are a major source of androgen, thought by many researchers to be the hormone most responsible for the libido, or sex drive, causing both increased susceptibility to psycho-sexual stimulation, and increased sensitivity of the external genitals. Estrogen replacement does not affect androgen level.

Androgens are produced in the adrenals, but also in the ovaries. Removing the adrenals causes changes similar to those experienced by some women after ovariectomy: diminished physical sensation and reduced response to stimulation. Androgen replacement has not generally been suggested by doctors, perhaps because of "masculinizing" changes such as a lowering of the voice and an increase in body hair.

Some doctors are now prescribing androgen pellets, inserted under the skin, with apparently good results. Women who have used the pellets successfully say they make a great difference in their sexual response. Ethel is fifty-five and for seven years had great difficulty after hysterectomy.

> When a friend finally told me about the androgen pellets and I got my doctor to find out how to get them, my sex life got better for the first time. They have made all the difference to me.

Other women are concerned about possible dangers of any kind of hormone artificially introduced into the woman's system. Janice is forty-two and has also had sexual difficulties.

> It's tempting to try to take another drug to help my sex life. But I just don't want to experiment anymore. I'm going to keep trying the healthful approaches and keep working on having a better sex life on my own. I'm just too scared to try a drug like that.

Since the prescription for home-brew estrogen also strengthens the adrenals, following that prescription should provide gentle stimulation of libido.

In addition to these anatomical phenomena, other changes in sexuality may be anticipated. After ovariectomy, even if you take estrogen, there are no monthly hormonal cycles. If you have had times of the month when you were more aroused and less aroused, those peaks and valleys will be evened out. Your hormonal balance will be most similar to that just before your period.

Oral estrogen, as well as hormonal changes, can cause shifts in the vaginal pH or the acid level in the vagina. This can lead to frequent yeast infections, or monilia, because the yeast grows more readily in a less acid vagina. Vaginitis, while it does not prevent sexual activity, can certainly diminish sexual pleasure. (If you do find recurring yeast infections after ovariectomy, see the next chapter. It could be that your sugar consumption is the culprit.)

The production of sexual odors and the response to the sexual smells may be affected by the hormone level. Animal research has documented the importance of sexual odors, or pheromones, in sexual behavior of animals. Castration of female animals substantially reduces the odors those animals produce, and the behavior of males toward castrated females is like the behavior of males toward males. Castrated females are furthermore less aware of odors of males.

Are there human sex pheromones? Do humans produce sexual smells that others pick up? Some current research is documenting human pheromones. The most intriguing study collected vaginal discharge on tampons from women at various times of their monthly cycles. When women and men were asked to rate the "pleasantness" of the odors, the ratings followed the same curve as the fertility of the woman. That is, at the time of the month when women were most fertile, men and women perceived the odors as most pleasant.

It seems very likely that smell plays a part in human sexuality, even if it is unconscious. A woman whose ovaries had been removed would produce the smells associated with the least fertile period of the monthly cycle. Castrated women may at some very subconscious level be less attractive sexually and may be less responsive sexually than a woman with full hormone production.

This may sound bizarre, and you may have no awareness of any changes in sexual odors. But some women do.

One is Shelly, who said excitedly,

> Susanne, I can't believe I'm hearing you say that. I have noticed a change in sexual odors. It used to be that when I sat down these wonderful smells would come up toward me. I never used to like to wash after making love because I enjoyed the odors so much. And now I just don't notice them anymore.

Emma is twenty-six and her hysterectomy when she was twenty-four was for a precancerous condition.

> I find that it's hardest to be around women. I can notice the smell if someone has their period, and I can notice the smell if someone has just had sex. That's information that I don't want to have, since I don't have those smells myself anymore.

Estrogen or androgen replacement does moderate many of the changes I have just described, but it does not eliminate them. Articles implying that estrogen replacement makes everything exactly as before are misleading. No one tries to convince a diabetic that the insulin shots are exactly the same as the insulin produced naturally in the body. A diabetic knows that he or she must take care not to get out of balance and that the insulin simply moderates some of the changes. Even if menopause were an "estrogen deficiency disease" as some people try to portray it, taking estrogen could not totally prevent all changes or adjustments.

Second, estrogen replacement is generally pushed at the same time as the negative sexual changes are presented. Lanson, for example, paints a very negative picture of the effects of early menopause on sexuality, and immediately follows with the panacea of estrogen replacement. The major experts on sex and the older woman, Masters and Johnson, refer frequently to "adequate" replacement to prevent sexual changes for older women. Before he began his sex research, Dr. Masters published many articles suggesting very high doses of estrogen for older women. Masters and Johnson probably would recommend a level of estrogen replacement higher than many women, concerned about the dangers of ERT, choose to take.

Sexuality is part of relationships and is therefore related to whatever is happening in the relationship. Some women find that their partners' feelings about their surgery affect their recovery.

Lina is a French woman of fifty-three.

> Sex? It's *comédie*! I act! That's all it is! I act! I used to be so passionate, always doing every little thing to please him and to please me. Now I have no interest at all. But I am afraid, afraid he will leave me for another woman.
>
> I did not tell him my ovaries were taken. He knows I had a hysterectomy, but if I tell him he will think I am castrated and no good.

After a couple more glasses of white wine Lina confided with bright eyes,

> I think I should have an affair! An affair with someone who doesn't know, just to make me happy. I want so much to be good for my husband, but I just can't.

Mary is thirty-five now. Her hysterectomy and ovariectomy were five years ago. She is one of the women who has described sexual changes.

> It's real crazy-making. I notice how I'm different. But I still think that I'm fine compared to other women. My husband and I have a real hard time. I was so quick to get turned on

that we never thought much about foreplay. Now it seems like a big burden, and he's not very interested in "working" at it. And I get upset because I'm not performing like I was before and don't want to even start out. We've had plenty of problems between us, and it may be all that, but I certainly notice a physical change.

Be sure not to let on who I am or what city you met me in, but I've had other lovers. That helps a lot, because with them I haven't been married for twelve years and I don't have children or household jobs on my mind. I still notice the physical changes, though, and it's upsetting to me. Also, I don't have much inclination for sex even though I know that when sex is good it relaxes my shoulders and makes me feel better all over. My husband says I'm sexless. I know I'm not, but with him I am more. The extra work to get turned on and the longer time to orgasm and the smaller orgasms really do make a difference with us.

Let's move to the brighter side. So far I've been describing changes that can affect sexuality in a negative way after hysterectomy or ovariectomy. Don't forget that these changes will be slight or unnoticeable to many of us, though they will be strongly felt by others of us. If your condition before your hysterectomy has significantly interfered with your sexual activity, the hysterectomy will provide overall relief. A severe pelvic infection or endometriosis, for example, can cause extreme pain from the thrusting of a penis. If your uterus is infected, orgasm itself can be very painful, even from masturbation or other kinds of sexual stimulation.

You may have a hysterectomy for fibroids, which can cause excessive bleeding. If you prefer to avoid sexual activity while you are menstruating, your opportunities for sex will no longer be limited after hysterectomy. You may be fatigued and anemic from heavy bleeding. Your hysterectomy may revive your general energy level and thus your general interest in sex.

Edie's hysterectomy was when she was forty-one. Her ovaries were not removed. She says,

> I was the Kotex Company's favorite customer. Before my hysterectomy . . . I went through a lot of stuff. Soiled sheets, soiled clothes, it was a whole big scene when my period rolled around. After my hysterectomy I *just* didn't have to worry about sleeping with a man, and checking his sheets every time I got up. So I guess what I'm trying to say is that my hysterectomy affected my relationships in a very positive way. Positive, meaning that I wasn't so anxious all the time. The only thing that changed my relationships with men after my hysterectomy was the fact that I was more sexually active and appreciative. I mean, think of it, because I was "fixed," I don't ever have to worry about getting pregnant. It's wonderful. I can enjoy myself to the fullest extent (before I couldn't do that) sexually.

Louise is fifty-nine and the mother of two grown daughters. She has been married for the past thirty-five years. She says there was a definite improvement in sexuality after the hysterectomy.

> When we were first married we used a diaphragm, and after the children were born we used a condom. My husband convinced me that the surgery would not have any effect on me as a woman or on my femininity or sexual desires. I had also read this in magazines and I believed it. For many years of my marriage, however, I did not particularly enjoy sex. I felt I had a low sex drive. But after the hysterectomy, particularly after starting to take Premarin, which helped with the vaginal problems I was experiencing, my interest in sex increased. I feel my relationship with my husband is better now than it has ever been. We have more sex play and more frequent intercourse. I was always a very nervous and tense person but now I am much more relaxed.

For many of us contraception is a great problem. After hysterectomy we never need to worry about whether the condom will break or the contraceptive foam has lost its power. Sex need not be interrupted to insert a diaphragm or use a condom. You don't need to worry about whether the Pill or IUD is going to harm your health. (Of course, for many of us the IUD has caused our hysterectomies and so not having to worry now is slightly ironic.)

Gladys, for example, was thirty-eight at the time of her hysterectomy.

> I can't tell you how much better sex is since I don't have to worry about being pregnant. The best thing about being pregnant and nursing had always been not having periods and not having to worry about pregnancy. Now I have that all the time. I feel like a new woman!

The beneficial effects of the reduction in pain sometimes do not appear immediately. Nancy's hysterectomy followed several years of extreme pelvic pain that eventually became so severe it required emergency surgery, when it was discovered that she had cancer. She says,

> I had never had intercourse without pain because I started having intercourse in 1968, which was when the pain started. So one would think it would be better and of course it was—the actual present moment of no pain was better than pain—but the fear of pain was so entrenched that it might as well have been there. I have only recently gotten to the point where I can relax and not be terrified of something coming into my abdomen. Now it's going to start getting better.

RESEARCH ON WOMEN'S PERCEPTIONS

What changes in sexuality do women actually notice after hysterectomy or ovariectomy?

Here is the summary. Approximately 60 percent of women report that sex is the same or better; approximately 40 percent say they have decreased sexual response after hysterectomy. The following table, prepared by Edith Bjornson and published in Zussman et al., summarizes the studies.

There are problems with all the studies, however; in addition the results are often interpreted in a biased way by the original author.

Few studies ask all the appropriate questions in a supportive context without betraying significant biases on the part of the researcher.

The research context is not always conducive to frankness. How open do you think you would be in a follow-up interview with the doctor who did your surgery? A psychologist or psychiatrist might probe more for negative reactions, but many of us would not feel very comfortable in that setting either.

Questions about sexuality are typically part of an interview about emotional reactions to hysterectomy. There is usually only one question reported, such as: "Since the operation my sexual relations with my husband have been very much better . . . about the same . . . very much worse . . ." Some research reports only comments about sexuality brought up spontaneously by the person being interviewed. Since we are frequently very reluctant to talk about sex, this method presents problems. Some articles do not even make it clear whether the subjects' ovaries had been removed. The researchers typically seem to think that sexual functioning is totally psychological. Not all studies of psychological reaction to hysterectomy even discuss sexuality.

Thus, the brief-question approach seems inadequate at best.

CHANGES IN SEXUAL RESPONSE REPORTED BY WOMEN
FOLLOWING HYSTERECTOMY WITH OR WITHOUT OOPHORECTOMY

INVESTIGATORS	TOTAL HYSTERECTOMY WITHOUT OOPHORECTOMY			TOTAL HYSTERECTOMY WITH BILATERAL OOPHORECTOMY		
	No. cases	% with same or incr. response	% with decr. response	No. cases	% with same or incr. response	% with decr. response
1973 Richards	56	63	37	—	—	—
1975 Craig and Jackson	49	67	32	—	—	—
1975 Utian	18	67	33	18	61	39
1977 Dennerstein, et al.	—	—	—	89	63	37
1977 Chakravarti, et al.	—	—	—	100	54	46

It is not conducive to the atmosphere of trust that the typical woman needs in order to describe changes she might have noticed. The assumption also is that the only relevant female sexuality is heterosexual intercourse. In fact at least one study omitted from the tabulations about sexual adjustment any women who were unmarried! No questions were asked about changes in frequency or characteristics of sexual drive or activity, about masturbation, about changes in intensity or frequency of orgasm.

Another problem in the methods of the studies—even the better ones—is that they are retrospective. They ask women to recall changes, a method which can lead to experimenter bias.

The typical treatment of sexuality in these research studies probably reflects not only limited research techniques but also society's and the researchers' stereotyped attitudes about the purpose of women's sexuality. In her book for lay women Nancy Nugent follows her statement that "sexual gratification . . . is in no way affected by the surgical removal of the uterus" with ". . . removal of the uterus, even with the cervix, in no way distorts the anatomy so as to make intercourse impossible or even difficult." This is true, at least if the woman's surgeon does not make the thoughtless errors in repair that Masters and Johnson describe. But the message is that a woman's purpose is to function for a man.

Whenever a study or an author refers only to intercourse and not to the woman's orgasms or sexual feelings, it seems to me that the writer is assuming that the extent of women's sexual experience is to be *able* to have intercourse, with or without pleasure. Diana Scully and Pauline Bart, in a wonderful paper called "A Funny Thing Happened on the Way to the Orifice," have alerted us to the ways that gynecology textbooks continue to proclaim as fact the traditional stereotypes that the findings of Kinsey and Masters and Johnson contradict. They report:

> Eight (two-thirds of the books published from 1963 to 1972) continued to state, contrary to Masters and Johnson's findings, that the male sex drive was stronger; and half

(six) still maintained that procreation was the major function of sex for the female. Two said that most women were "frigid" and another stated that one-third were sexually unresponsive. Two repeated that the vaginal orgasm was the only mature response.

Two studies by women are exceptions to this rule. Gail Whitman, a graduate student, questioned women who had had radical pelvic surgery for cancer. Many of them had had almost all of their vagina removed and sometimes other parts of their sexual organs. She found that many women said they had "adequate sexual adjustment," but for many of them that meant that the man manipulated their genitals less and they manipulated the man's genitals more. This suggests that many women learn to subordinate their new sexual needs to satisfying their partner's.

Shere Hite's survey of women's sexual behavior shows the relatively minor role that intercourse plays in many women's sexual satisfaction.

For many women orgasms come from direct stimulation of their clitoris. Intercourse is a pleasurable (or tolerated) part of sex, but the major satisfaction comes from stroking with fingers or tongue. So when people try to understand women's feelings after hysterectomy based on asking whether they are able to have intercourse without pain, they cannot fully understand the hysterectomy experience. For other women, internal stimulation is most important, yet a question about intercourse without pain does not reflect their experiences either.

Even if researchers were to probe for more sexual data, many women might find it difficult to verbalize the effects of the subtle changes that do occur, especially to researchers who have not had hysterectomies. I like to use the parallel of body temperature. Some people are aware when their temperature is elevated, and some are not. Fever may affect their feelings and body processes in ways that they do not notice. It is illogical to assume that physiologically predictable changes that are not consciously noticed have no effect.

The impact of hysterectomy on men is generally not acknowledged. Sexual problems following hysterectomy are inevitably blamed on the woman, although there is evidence that men are very distressed by it. For women in heterosexual relationships at the time of the hysterectomy, the reactions of their male partners can significantly influence their sexual adjustment. Masters and Johnson indicate that the husband's reaction may be "the most important worry." A number of studies show male behavior to be a significant posthysterectomy problem. One authority advises physicians to "support, encourage, and counsel the woman's sexual partner, since he is potentially *our* greatest ally and *her* best therapist."

The tendency to attribute negative changes to the woman's poor psychological functioning, rather than to look at physical changes or at men's reactions to make a total picture, is also seen in the few studies in the literature that have in-depth interviews with women. In two major studies the few women who described sexual problems in some detail are not believed. Although they describe recognizable physical changes, their descriptions are interpreted as resulting from their emotional problems.

We must also examine the attitudes of doctors toward hysterectomy. Bernardine Paulshock, in a 1976 article in *Today's Health* quotes from the important gynecology textbook by Emil Novak: " '. . . no drastic results are found following the removal of the uterus. . . . Indeed, it should not be construed as callous if any gynecologists feel that, in the woman that has completed her family, the uterus is rather a worthless organ.' " Paulshock adds, "This is indeed the attitude of most gynecologists. While it may seem harsh and ill-phrased, it is a logical viewpoint and one with which I personally agree."

It is not surprising that writers who are convinced that hysterectomy has no psychological or sexual or physical effects should communicate that perception to their audience. To call it unbiased research and to encourage women to make major decisions with the idea that there will be no change is extremely misleading. Women considering hysterectomy need realistic discussion of the changes that could occur, so we can make an informed decision knowing some of the risks. We also need to know that whatever problems occur can be overcome.

CONSPIRACY OF SILENCE

Have you been told about all of these possible sexual changes after hysterectomy? Have you been informed of the implications of ovariectomy? I doubt it. A massive conspiracy of silence surrounds hysterectomy and its possible consequences. Contributing to the conspiracy are doctors, nurses, and counselors. They are often motivated by a concern that women not become inappropriately frightened, but the effect of this reticence is nevertheless to keep information hidden.

Writers and clinicians work especially hard to silence one source of information about hysterectomy: other women. They constantly warn against women talking with one another and sharing information about their experiences. Here are some examples, written by women (I am sorry to say) for the general public.

> So, do not listen to your bridge club or your bowling league. The women you speak with may have had a change in her sex life after hysterectomy: what she may not be telling you is that consciously or unconsciously she wanted it that way.

> It is sometimes hard to ignore folklore presented by a friend as fact, particularly if the friend has had similar surgery herself.

Even conversations with friends can be informative, although the prospective patient should be careful to shun old wives' tales that can feed fear and produce grotesque misconceptions about the aftermath of hysterectomy.

Nearly every article for lay women contains warnings against listening to "old wives' tales," that is, to other women's experiences. The lay press, in newspaper articles or pamphlets or books such as this, takes its share of beatings from some doctors also. This is an English comment:

> Erroneous notions about the effects of the operation are fostered by opinionated and ill-informed comment in the lay press. . . . Some of the poor results of hysterectomy can be directly attributed to the harmful effects of newspaper medicine.

The argument against women having information about hysterectomy before their surgery (or before their decision) is generally that if we know of possible risks, those problems will occur after surgery, because of our expectations. This is a very dangerous argument and also not supported by research evidence. The argument suggests that information should be kept from women for their own good, and that we should not be allowed to make a truly informed decision.

An article in the January 1979 issue of the *American Journal of Public Health* provides some evidence that it is not true that more information for consumers about drug side effects will lead to an unnecessary increase in symptoms. The implication for hysterectomy is that if women are told of possible side effects or sexual changes, symptoms may be more quickly noticed and reported so that treatment can begin and be more effective.

Women today are told of many of the changes that may occur during pregnancy and childbirth. We are not denied information because the information may cause morning sickness; rather, we are told ways to minimize morning sickness if it does occur.

We are told about changes that could affect our sexuality, so we can make the appropriate adjustment. We learn from other women the variety of childbirth experiences. Self-help groups, in which information about pregnancy and childbirth is shared, such as prepared childbirth classes, are encouraged.

With hysterectomy this information is withheld, and women are discouraged from learning about the changes other women have experienced. In the support groups that I have helped to establish, women are very skillful at distinguishing another woman's experience from their own.

The self-help movement in general has produced some extremely significant new thinking and new forms of health education.

Self-help groups in areas such as contraceptive information, mastectomy recovery, and pregnancy and childbirth are extremely effective forums for communicating good health information.

Even with all this emphasis on self-help, the medical profession continues to discourage women from learning more about their bodies. Two articles in the August 1978 *New England Journal of Medicine* document the improved detection of palpable breast nodules (lumps) by women who regularly practice breast self-examination. Despite these findings the same issue of the journal ran an editorial taking the position that the advantages of breast self-examination are questionable, and that physicians should remain hesitant about recommending this procedure to their patients.

We see more and more evidence to document the fact that the more informed patients are, the more effective is their health behavior. Yet in many ways, that increased information is discouraged. I wonder if this is a conscious or unconscious strategy to retain power in the hands of medical personnel. The more information we have, and the more assertive we are, the less power they have.

As regards hysterectomy, if the research studies do show that most women are happier after hysterectomy, why are medical people so concerned about our sharing information? One possible reason is that some misinformation is in fact communicated when women discuss their experiences. This is partly attributable to our health care system itself, which keeps information mysterious and available only through a rigid hierarchy.

In fact the information doctors themselves communicate is often very limited. Recently researchers investigating the language that physicians thought their patients knew found that patients understood far more than the physicians expected. Nevertheless, the physicians routinely used language with patients that they were convinced the patients did not understand. This makes us think that physicians typically underestimate the knowledge of patients and in addition are unwilling to communicate with patients. Consequently, if women in talking with each other do communicate incorrect information, the health system must take most of the blame.

There is a further explanation for the reluctance of doctors for women to share information about hysterectomy. Forty percent of women have sexual problems after hysterectomy. If that fact were widely known, many women would hesitate to have a hysterectomy. Since doctors tend to recommend hysterectomy quite lightly, they also tend to minimize its risks. Women may communicate much more negative information about hysterectomy than the doctors wish.

IT'S ALL IN YOUR HEAD

One of the most infuriating attitudes taken by doctors and writers is that any problems a woman might have after a hysterectomy are psychogenic, that is, caused by emotional dislocations. At some level I do believe this is true. Our minds and our bodies are much more interdependent than either psychologists or doctors have been taught to perceive. In a certain way we are in charge of what happens in our bodies, and illnesses or physical problems do have a particular meaning and a particular function for us.

All the resources, information, and healers that are linked under the umbrella of holistic medicine emphasize that relationship. Holistic health people are developing an understanding of depression and mental illness as an allergy or biochemical response. Holistic health workers are also using mental powers to heal illnesses as severe as cancer.

Some day our health system will be integrated enough so that the connection between our bodies and our minds will be understood. In the meantime I am very suspicious when I hear people talking about psychogenic disorders. Typically they deny physical or organic causes for a complaint and attribute it to the woman's mental state. The medical profession commonly thinks of several problems of women as psychogenic and treats them with psychoactive drugs, despite evidence that suggests the problems are organic. Premenstrual pain, nausea of pregnancy, pain in labor, and colic in babies are all examples of such problems. These problems are always treated by psychological drugs or ineffective counseling, whereas if the problem were seen as organic, more effective treatment would be used. This may well be a manifestation of sexual prejudice.

A recent survey of doctors presented them with a set of symptoms and asked them to describe the treatments they would recommend. When the symptoms were presented by men, the doctors typically suggested a medical drug or surgery treatment. When the symptoms were presented by women, the doctors typically assumed the symptoms were psychological and prescribed tranquilizers.

Effects of hysterectomy on sexuality have the same characteristics. Hysterectomy causes a great many changes in the physiology of sexuality. Ovariectomy causes even more. Hysterectomy also has an important symbolic meaning. Sexuality is dependent on both physical and psycho-social factors. When sexuality after hysterectomy is discussed, however, the physical changes seem to be ignored and only the symbolic and psychosocial ones are considered.

Masters and Johnson take two positions on this, depending on their audience. Discussing postsurgical dyspareunia (painful intercourse) in *Human Sexual Inadequacy*, they stress that they always believe and investigate reports of pain. "If a woman complains of pain with intercourse, her complaint is accepted at face value, and steps are taken to identify the biophysical source of the coital distress. The diagnosis of psychosomatic dyspareunia . . . must be made by exclusion."

To the readers of *Redbook* magazine, Masters and Johnson say something different. "However, if a woman discovers, for example, that after the surgery she doesn't lubricate as well as she did before, you can be sure that as soon as she brings this to the attention of her physician he or she will look beyond the hysterectomy for other causes of the problem, and it is far and away the best bet that the symptoms will turn out to be psychosomatic."

In their writing about female sexuality Masters and Johnson stress that for women the psychosocial influences can be very crucial in sexual experience. Many writers point to these statements to defend their assertion that sexual problems following hysterectomy are due to psychological factors. Masters and Johnson's statement should be interpreted to mean that physical difficulties can frequently be overcome because people do have cognitive capabilities. The statement is usually interpreted only to mean that psychological factors can cause sexual problems. The physical nature of sexual changes must be acknowledged, not to say that those changes will make sexuality impossible, but to say there may be changes that influence sexual activity and feelings and that can be dealt with.

Not acknowledging physical changes leads to inadequate help for the woman with problems. For problems of lubrication, for example, lubricating jelly is suggested, but often not with full understanding that lubrication is more than wetness: it is the first indication of arousal. Lubricating jelly certainly should help to make penetration less painful if the woman is not aroused, but is that the situation writers and doctors should encourage? Lubricating jelly may also make clitoral stimulation less painful, so that the woman can be aroused and her natural lubrication started. But lubrication is similar to erection, and suggesting that jelly can adequately replace it is to ignore its physiological function.

Also, lower androgen level may decrease libido and orgasms may depend heavily on internal sensations.

Not acknowledging physical changes also communicates the impression that if a woman does have problems, it is due to her own poor adjustment. Since sex is seen as psychological, if she has difficulty the explanation must lie in her own personal inability to cope. She may feel she must have been "too attached" to her childbearing function, deserving the "punishment" of sexual problems.

Many women try very hard to take responsibility for their sexuality and to deal with any changes they have noticed on an emotional level. Phyllis is now thirty-eight, and her hysterectomy and ovariectomy were five years ago.

> I've been in therapy and I'm seeing a lot more clearly the way that I may have been mixed up about my femininity all along. But I still notice the physical changes that you talk about, and the therapy hasn't helped that.

Jean was thirty at the time of her hysterectomy and ovariectomy.

> The man I was living with left me soon after my surgery. I guess I haven't dealt with those feelings enough, because I am less interested in sex than I had been.

Gloria, forty-three, says,

> I take estrogen, and have for three years. I use lubricating jelly. But sex still isn't the same. It must be my emotions,

though everything is wonderful in all the other parts of my life. It's not that sex is terrible for me, it just isn't the same. Maybe a few more years of therapy will help.

For each of these women a physical explanation of her experience is very helpful.

The tendency to assess women in an either narrowly psychological or physical way can be seen in the contrast with comparable discussions of men. Orchiectomy, removing the testicles, is parallel to ovariectomy. "The generally accepted opinions are that bilateral orchiectomy without testosterone supplements will lead to impotency." Yet ovariectomy is assumed to cause minor, surmountable problems, and most difficulties are thought to be psychogenic. Here, the same physical event for men is assumed to cause enormous sexual problems and for women it is assumed to cause minor sexual problems, and then only if the woman's adjustment is less than adequate.

Another example is in the contrast between treatments for men and for women in the middle years. There is great controversy in thinking about treating women in the middle years. Some doctors believe there are few physical problems and treat menopausal women with tranquilizers. Other doctors believe menopause represents a major hormonal imbalance and treat menopausal women with long-term estrogen. When men are in the middle years, called the climacteric, however, physicians typically test men carefully for both physical and psychological causes before treating any of the problems a man may have. Women need to be thought about as individuals also. Some problems may be psychological, and some may be physical. Doctors need to think carefully about each person rather than assuming a general form of treatment for menopause.

It is ironic to look at the contrast in thinking about the effect of ovariectomy or hysterectomy on sexuality today compared to one hundred years ago. Then, hysterectomy and especially ovariectomy were common treatments for "excessive" sexuality.

Today doctors need to justify the very high rate of hysterectomy. Because "good sexual adjustment" is considered extremely important for women, doctors now assure them there will be no change in sexuality after hysterectomy, and little change after castration. Notice the way medical ideology adjusts to the needs of the surgeon!

TAKING CHARGE

If you have noticed changes in your sexual feelings since your hysterectomy, know that you are not alone. Your body has had some major changes, and those changes have had an effect. You are also in charge of your sexuality, though, and here are some strategies for assuring a happy sex life after hysterectomy.

Try to develop sources of support, places where you can express your fears and feelings without judgment. As I have said elsewhere, I find re-evaluation co-counseling to be an excellent source of support. A co-counselor will assist you in getting to the tears you need to shed or the fear or rage you need to express in order to heal the hurts and move on from there. A co-counselor will also remind you of how very well you are in fact doing. One phrase a co-counselor might ask you to repeat is the phrase "I am fully female." For all women that phrase brings up many feelings, but for women after hysterectomy it brings up a particular kind of grief. Using a phrase like that as a shortcut to express feelings can assist us in moving rapidly to better functioning.

Another kind of support can be found in a group of women who have had hysterectomies. Of course you will respect one another's experiences and assume that another woman may have noticed fewer or greater changes than you have. But there will certainly be women who express feelings similar to your own, and that can be extremely helpful.

If you do notice changes in lubrication, a lubricant like K-Y jelly or scented oils can feel very good, especially as your clitoris is stroked. It can help in the transition to arousal. K-Y jelly is a lubricating jelly such as doctors use when they do a pelvic examination, and you can buy it in a drugstore. Jelly can help with clitoral stroking but some women find oils work better for vaginal penetration. Do not use Vaseline in your vagina or any other interior part of your body. Vaseline is a petroleum product and is not absorbed by your body. Scented oils such as those used in massage can be very pleasant. Some women prefer to use wheat germ oil, vitamin E oil, or apricot-kernel oil, which have some properties similar to estrogen.

Of course, you can take estrogen by mouth or use estrogen cream to moderate some of the dryness. The estrogen cream should not be used specifically as a lubricant when having sex, but should be used once or twice a week as a suppository. Estrogens, even taken vaginally, have major health hazards.

An excellent physical therapy for vaginal dryness is masturbation and lovemaking. Not only does it reassure us and our partners that we are all right, it also has a direct beneficial effect on our hormones and sexual tissue. For many of us, the more frequently we are aroused, the more quickly we will become lubricated.

But many women, and many men, find it difficult to establish a satisfying sex life after hysterectomy. In fact, with the excessive emphasis on sexuality plus the constraints most of us grew up with about feeling good about our bodies, many women find a satisfying sex life hard to reach in any circumstance. There are increasing numbers of resources available for women to help themselves to enjoy their bodies more. A good example is *For Yourself: The Fulfillment of Female Sexuality,* by Lonnie Garfield Barbach, Ph.D. Barbach is a sex therapist who leads the reader very gently through exercises exploring their bodies and gives the reader permission to enjoy touching and pleasuring themselves. She presents exercises that can be done with a partner to gradually reduce some of the impediments to good sexual expression together.

After reading one of the helpful books on sexual expression, you may consider sex therapy, alone or preferably with your partner. It can be very helpful. Generally you can arrange for a limited number of sessions.

When I have spoken of women and their partners, you may be assuming that I am speaking only of women and men. Women who relate sexually with other women also have hysterectomies (possibly less often, since hysterectomy is sometimes a complication of contraception). From lesbian women I have talked with I have heard a similar variety of stories about feelings after hysterectomy. It is a big event, support is needed, and it can have effects on a woman's feelings about herself or on her partner's feelings. Most lesbian women feel much better after hysterectomy, just as heterosexual women do.

Some women who have related to men and women find that making love with women, since it is often slower and less intercourse-centered, is more satisfying. Some find the site of their orgasm transfers from internal to clitoral. I hope we see society changing so that loving relationships between women are more acknowledged and visible. For many of us, women are our closest friends, and since most married women will be widows, we may spend many years without an intimate relationship. Maggie Kuhn of the Gray Panthers has pointed out that loving and intimate relationships between women are a way to fulfill our needs as we grow older. It is also a way to keep our sexual organs functioning well.

The challenge of overcoming sexual changes after hysterectomy can seem overwhelming, but many women find that they grow from meeting and overcoming the challenges. We are in charge of our sexuality.

Chapter Nine

HOME-BREW ESTROGEN

My doctor gave me a shot of DES in the hospital and I have been taking Premarin ever since. I love it! When I don't take it, I feel terrible. Those little pills really have saved my life.

I can't take estrogen because they say my cancer may have been caused by hormones I took before. It's awful! I wake up in the night drenched.

I'm taking Premarin but I'm really worried. I don't like taking anything foreign in my body, especially a hormone that might cause cancer. But I don't know how to get off it.

Estrogen replacement therapy certainly is controversial. Estrogens are dangerous drugs commonly prescribed for women at menopause. ERT will also probably be prescribed to any woman who has a surgical menopause with hysterectomy. Estrogens can reduce or eliminate hot flashes, and they help relieve vaginal dryness. They may possibly have some relationship to whether a woman gets osteoporosis, or brittle bones. As short-term medication they can help a woman through a transitional time. Many doctors, however, prescribe large doses of estrogen whether or not a woman has troublesome symptoms. Many women take it for a very long time. If you have a premature menopause, you may be advised to take estrogen even longer than a woman might at menopause.

Sandra, who is now thirty-five, spoke up in a meeting.

> Help through a transition? My ovaries were out when I was twenty-nine. My doctor then and doctors since then have said I should take estrogen for twenty years until I would have menopause normally. I can't help but worry, whichever way I go. If I don't take it I worry about my bones, if I do take it I worry about cancer.

Sandra puts it in a nutshell. The estrogen controversy is bad enough for women in a normal menopause, but for women whose menopause occurs very early it is even more confusing.

Estrogen replacement therapy can take several forms. Conjugated equine estrogens are made to be chemically like the urine of pregnant mares. Premarin is the major brand (get it? pregnant mares) and it is made by Ayerst Laboratories. Other estrogen products such as DES (diethylstilbestrol) or Estrone, may be prescribed. You might take ERT as tablets, as an injection, or as a vaginal cream. Sometimes estrogen by mouth causes nausea, so the injection is used. Sometimes progestin is given in conjunction with estrogen. This is to further "simulate" the natural hormone balance. It is supposed to prevent "unopposed estrogen," which may cause some of the problems associated with estrogen.

DANGERS OF ESTROGEN

Why is there a controversy about estrogen? Estrogens have been shown repeatedly to be related to increased incidence of endometrial cancer, gallbladder disease, and possibly also breast cancer. Endometrial cancer occurs more often in women taking estrogen than in women who do not take estrogen. If you look at the whole society, both the number of prescriptions for estrogen and the number of cases of cancer of the endometrium rose steadily until 1976, and since then both have declined at the same rate. Looking at the rates of endometrial cancer for post-menopausal women, among women who do not take estrogen the rate is approximately one per one thousand postmenopausal women per year. After two to four years of use of estrogens, the rate increases several-fold. The risk of endometrial cancer increases the longer the estrogen is used, and the risk declines after the estrogen is discontinued. The statistics suggest, however, that although the rate of cancer of the endometrium has gone up, the number of women who die from the disease has not increased. This may be because of early detection with regular Pap smears.

For all of these statistics, of course, there are real women and real grief.

> Fifteen years ago when I was thirty-eight my doctor said "I can make you beautiful forever. I can keep you young and looking beautiful." Of course I did it. I took the estrogen because I did not want to grow old and wrinkled. Then one year ago I am in for a checkup and bang. I have cancer and he says I have to have a hysterectomy. This doctor says it is from taking the estrogen. And I have been depressed, very depressed.

Cystic hyperplasia of the endometrium results in the spotting or staining or "breakthrough bleeding" that women sometimes experience in menopause or when taking estrogen. Hyperplasia is excessive overgrowth of normal tissue. Cystic hyperplasia is considered a premalignant condition, and it has been shown to be associated with "unopposed estrogen." Unopposed estrogen means that your body contains estrogen but not progesterone, another hormone that is part of the menstrual cycle. Unopposed estrogen can exist if a woman is not ovulating, or if she takes estrogen medication. It is very important to have a checkup if you ever have unexplained bleeding. You should probably have a suction curettage, or a D & C, to determine the nature of the endometrium and to rule out cancer. Some experts suggest that even if you do not have abnormal bleeding, your uterine lining should be checked every year if you are taking estrogen.

Some doctors prescribe progestins for several days of each month if a woman is taking estrogen. This has been shown to reduce the likelihood of endometrial hyperplasia. For that reason it may also reduce the risk of developing cancer of the endometrium. However, many doctors are very concerned about widespread use of progestins before the risks of these drugs are thoroughly evaluated. We could very easily have another DES story or another Premarin story, where women take drugs for many years and then discover later what the risks have been.

This information often provokes a lively exchange:

> Wait a second, Susanne! You're talking about cancer of the endometrium, but I don't have any endometrium! That's part of the uterus isn't it?

> Well, it's relevant to me! That's why I'm having this hysterectomy, for endometrial cancer. That doctor who put me on estrogen—I'm so mad at him I could throw him across the room.

> I'm worried about my mother. I won't get endometrial cancer, but my mother takes estrogen and her doctor tells

her that since she takes progestin she doesn't have anything to worry about. Are you saying she does?

I can't believe that endometrial cancer is the only danger. Come on, Susanne, get on with it. Tell us the rest.

Yes, there is more. Not only are there additional risks, but statements about progestin's safety are seriously challenged.

Breast cancer remains a concern. In experimental animals researchers have definitely shown an association between estrogens and breast cancer. Such a relationship has not been proven in humans, although there is cause for alarm. One major study showed a 30 percent increase in breast cancer in postmenopausal women who were using high-dose estrogen.

Premarin-type estrogens have been implicated in serious gallbladder diseases also. One study showed that a woman taking estrogens ran a risk of gallbladder disease two and one half times higher than if she were not taking estrogens. Experimental studies show that estrogens can affect the production of lithogenous bile, possibly promoting the production of gallstones.

WHY ARE SO MANY ESTROGENS PRESCRIBED?

One reason is that doctors are trained to prescribe medications fairly freely. Today's holistic health movement is challenging many of the assumptions that drugs are good for you and that good care automatically includes use of drugs. But most doctors are trained to see a symptom and think of a drug that would relieve that symptom. A prescription for home-brew estrogen would be far harder to write, since it involves a very general change in life habits. In addition, most of the changes would be outside the jurisdiction of the doctor, so the doctor would not be paid.

Doctors say the reason so many estrogens are prescribed is that women request them. Of course women request them! From the 1966 book by Robert A. Wilson called *Feminine Forever* and David Reuben's *Everything You Always Wanted to Know About Sex* . . . , which present a very negative (and false) picture of menopause, women learned to seek estrogens as a magical treatment to prevent aging and preserve youthfulness. Those claims sounded attractive to us, because youth is so valued in our society. More recently, *The Lila Nachtigall Report* presents a modified but still very pro-estrogen picture.

All of these books have been seriously criticized scientifically for their research methods and by social critics for their extremely stereotyped picture of older women. But the damage is done. Our public libraries have those books, and they do not have the criticisms, which appear in more obscure journals. Only with books like Rosetta Reitz's *Menopause: A Positive Approach*, and Barbara and Gideon Seaman's *Women and the Crisis in Sex Hormones* do women get a different picture of menopause and find support for going to their doctor and saying, "I have hot flashes but I don't want to take estrogen for the rest of my life. What should I do?" It has not been easy for women to go against the prevailing prejudices in favor of medicine and against older women.

One encouragement to both doctors' prescribing habits and women's requests is the marketing efforts of the makers of estrogen drugs. The advertising strategy for estrogen replacement therapy drugs capitalizes on the negative image of older women. The Seamans in *Women and the Crisis in Sex Hormones* describe several ads for ERT products.

> A recent ad for one E.R.T. product, Ogen, depicts a woman dressed for travel and clutching a Delta Airline ticket, but

unable to get up from her chair. Her impatient husband stands behind her, glaring at his watch. "Bon Voyage?" says the copy. "Suddenly she'd rather not go. She's waited 30 years for this trip. Now she just doesn't have the 'bounce.' She has headaches, hot flashes, and she feels tired and nervous all of the time. And for no reason at all she cries."
Another E.R.T. ad states unblushingly: "For the menopausal symptoms that bother *him* most." Again we see a drab and unattractive woman, with her victimized husband standing by. . . .
[A Premarin ad depicts a harpy.] The copy states: "Almost any tranquilizer might calm her down . . . but at her age, estrogen may be what she really needs." As there is no valid medical evidence that estrogen improves mental outlook, the ad cites patients' testimonials: "Patients taking Premarin alone often report relief of emotional symptoms due to estrogen deficiency . . . and an improved sense of well-being."

These advertisements reinforce social stereotypes of older women and teach doctors to prescribe drugs for any problems the woman—or her husband or the doctor—might have.

Ayerst and companies like it have "created" menopause as an "estrogen deficiency disease." What a terrific marketing strategy! A new disease, which will be experienced by every woman, is invented and a drug produced to "treat" it.

A market as lucrative as that must be protected at all costs. As the evidence linking estrogen to cancer was being published, the Ayerst company sent reassuring letters to all doctors. They hired a public relations firm, Hill and Knowlton, to provide advice about protecting their market from the publicity about the dangers of estrogen. *Majority Report*, a major women's newspaper, published a letter from Hill and Knowlton to Ayerst recommending activities to prevent the loss of sales, including:

Placing articles on menopause in major women's magazines
Placing syndicated columnists on women's pages

Articles in general magazines
Contacting science editors
A film on the menopause, etc.

The scary thing here is that it is hard enough to figure out whether or not to take a drug when there are reasons for taking it and dangers are involved. When the manufacturers of the drug deliberately take steps to prevent new information from having any impact on their sales, it is very alarming. People can be good health care consumers only with full information.

The marketing activities by Ayerst prompted a complaint by Ralph Nader's Health Research Group to the Food and Drug Administration. A new package-insert is now required. Try to find it in a package of Premarin. It is your right as a consumer to have the package insert. You will see that it has very strong information about the possible hazards of estrogen drugs. The insert also specifically denies some of the earlier claims made by Ayerst for estrogen.

Articles showing the relationship of estrogen use to endometrial cancer began appearing in the most prestigious medical journals as early as 1975. Consumer activists picked up on the research studies and began to publicize the results to consumers and legislators. Newsletters and journals for women and for older people carried articles warning of the dangers of estrogen. Governments at the state and federal level held policy hearings, and the Food and Drug Administration invited testimony about estrogen drugs. The new package-insert was forced on Ayerst Laboratories by the federal regulation agencies. Research about the risks had been published for several years, and yet the company itself made no effort to modify their promotion until forced.

All of us who are involved in the women's health movement, and that includes you, can take pride in the new consumer information about estrogens. You should know that the rate of new cases of endometrial cancer leveled off as evidence of the dangers of estrogen became known.

HOME-BREW ESTROGEN

Estrogen is a dangerous drug. Yet we often have distressing symptoms either around the time of menopause or if our ovaries have been removed. I wish I could suggest a magic alternative. But the trouble with the hormone-like drugs is that they are magic bullets. They help relieve certain symptoms but cause other unknown effects. We need to learn other ways to help our bodies be healthier and symptom-free.

The ovaries are not the only source of estrogen in the female body. There are cases of women well into their eighties whose bodies show a measurable amount of estrogen. This estrogen is referred to technically as "endogenous estrogen." I like to call it "home-brew estrogen." We make it ourselves, it's not exactly like store-bought, and it works very well.

HOME-BREW ESTROGEN RECIPE

The recipe for home-brew estrogen consists of a series of steps. Each of us needs to take two steps toward better health in all the major areas. You probably know what the next step for you is, and if you need information, any of the books on healthful living can be helpful. The recipe is free-form and goes like this:

EXERCISE

Take, one at a time, two steps toward a better exercise program for you. That might include doing some exercise every day, or it might include adding stretching exercises to walking you already do, or it might include regular running in addition to the stretching or walking you already do. To help produce the home-brew estrogen, you need to improve your exercise program.

NUTRITION

Take two steps toward better nutrition. A good first step for many of us is to eliminate sugar and foods containing sugar. A second step might be to make sure you have fresh fruits and vegetables one more time per day than previously, or to make sure you consume some dairy products each day.

BEVERAGES

Take one step toward reducing your consumption of alcoholic beverages and beverages containing caffeine.

SUPPLEMENTS

Review your vitamin and mineral supplement program and improve it. This may mean beginning to take supplements, or it may mean considering additional supplements.

SEXUAL ACTIVITY

Pursue regular sexual activity leading to orgasm and be more active than you have been. This could mean engaging in more sexual activity by yourself, or it could mean a conscious effort to pursue sexual activity with someone else more frequently.

That is the prescription. True, it is easier to take a pill. But the pill will not do nearly as much for us as this prescription will. The pill also may cause problems that we know about now or that may surprise us later.

HORMONES AND HOME-BREW ESTROGEN

There is no unchallenged explanation for endogenous estrogen. It may be that the traditional medical understanding has been based on assumptions limited by stereotypes: stereotypes about the differences between women and men and stereotypes about the relationships between body and mind.

According to some explanations estrogen and other hormones are produced in the ovaries and other sites, primarily the adrenals. Others say that the ovaries and adrenals produce precursors to estrogen and the estrogen is actually produced in fatty tissue under the skin. In any case, it seems far more complex than a simple model in which a drug could truly be the same as the natural process. Drugs are taken by mouth or injection, and all at once, rather than in the fluctuating natural rhythm.

There is some evidence that weight is a factor and heavier women make more estrogen. Heavier women are more subject to estrogen-related diseases such as breast cancer, but less subject to diseases associated with low estrogen level, like osteoporosis. It is possible that a higher level of home-brew estrogen may be a factor in those relationships.

Whatever your body weight, it appears that the adrenal gland must be functioning well in order for the home-brew estrogen to be produced. Even before menopause very small amounts of estrogen and other sex hormones are produced in the adrenals. After a normal, healthy menopause the hormones produced by the adrenals are relatively more important than those produced by the ovaries. In a normal menopause the ovaries gradually reduce the production of hormones and the home-brew estrogen continues to be produced by the adrenal.

After ovariectomy, of course, the hormones produced by the ovaries are gone. The only remaining estrogen is produced by the adrenals. Surgery being an enormous stress, the adrenals are probably less able to function than they normally are. No wonder our bodies are thrown into a tizzy! Dr. Kurt W. Donsbach in a booklet called *Hysterectomy* says,

> 1.   The ovaries have been surgically removed; 2.   There has been a sudden or instant cessation of ovarian hormonal activity, instant menopause; 3.   The thyroid and adrenal glands had no warning that such would happen, as would occur in a natural menopause; 4.   Such a reaction is a severe stress which shows itself in a strained reaction of the adrenal cortex; 5.   Also, the thyroid is stressed so that it may and probably will work abnormally for a period of time.

To make home-brew estrogen we need to help our adrenal gland function at its utmost. Since the adrenals are the parts of our bodies that help deal with stress, it seems logical that we should reduce the stress that our bodies need to deal with.

HOME-BREW ESTROGEN AND STRESS REDUCTION

What kinds of stress should we reduce in order to assist our adrenals and thus assist the production of home-brew estrogen? First, many substances we eat are very stressful to our bodies. If we do not ask our bodies to deal with substances such as alcohol, sugar, salt, and coffee, we will be enduring much less stress. Not only will that make us feel better, function better, and rest better, but also it will free our adrenal gland from dealing with some of the stress and strengthen it for helping to produce more home-brew estrogen.

Sugar appears to play an especially key role here. Many women have said to me that they perceive hot flashes to be connected with sudden changes in blood-sugar level. Some of us find that if we eat too much sugar or drink alcohol, we get hot sweats, even if we are not postmenopausal. For postmenopausal women, it seems to happen even more.

There is research suggesting that the explanation for hot flashes as results of fluctuating blood sugar is as plausible as the explanation that hot flashes are caused by low estrogen. One of the indirect effects of estrogen drugs is to raise the blood-sugar level, so Premarin may prevent hot flashes by artificially masking the symptoms of an underlying nutritional problem. Another cause of hot flashes could be stress, which stimulates an output of adrenaline. Giving estrogen drugs without removing the original cause of the stress further weakens the adrenals.

The significance of this for avoiding estrogen replacement therapy is that if we cut sugar and foods containing refined sugar out of our diet, we will probably feel fewer of the symptoms of low estrogen level. We will probably feel a lot better too!

Many of us have come to this information in a variety of ways by ourselves. In a talk I gave recently an attractive, relaxed, gray-haired woman spoke.

> I was having a lot of trouble with hot flashes and generally feeling bad after my hysterectomy. My doctor put me on a hypoglycemia diet. I have to eat high protein, low carbo-hydrate meals frequently. Since I have been eating that way, I feel much better and I don't get hot flashes.

Sally, a librarian, wrote to me from Princeton, New Jersey:

> I do have hypoglycemia and have known it since 1972 and have been on the traditional high protein, low carbohydrate diet. My last glucose tolerance test though, in January, was much worse than my three previous ones, and I wonder if the hysterectomy didn't throw me farther off balance. My former boss says he developed hypoglycemia after a serious

operation. Any research on this? At any rate eating a high protein snack before bed had virtually eliminated waking up with a headache.

The bad effects of coffee are notorious, and getting off it can be a liberation. Madeline shared her amazement:

> I am appalled at the changes I noticed two days after quitting coffee, and I was only drinking four to six cups a day. I had been seeing a chiropractor for extreme pain in my neck and terrible headaches—that is gone! I've had diarrhea for two years—that's gone. I'd been bloated and gassy and thought it was food allergies. And I don't get the hunger for sweets in the afternoon. I truly don't believe it!

In addition to the stress caused by the substances that we ingest, living in our society produces many kinds of stress. Women have extremely stressful lives, with many conflicting role expectations. Women in the menopause face special stress. Middle age is thought to be a time when women's usefulness is outlived. The negative stereotypes about middle-aged women could fill several pages—try it! We are told that without childbearing capacity our worth as people diminishes. If you think about it, many of the symptoms of low estrogen are also symptoms of stress and probably of adrenal weakness.

Those of us who have had a hysterectomy have experienced the enormous stress of major surgery. Our bodies require far more healing than is generally realized to recover fully from a major operation. Also, most of us had been ill before the hysterectomy. Thus, our reserves of home-brew estrogen had probably been depleted before we ever went into surgery.

Women learn an enormous variety of ways to cope with stress. Some join a yoga class. This provides a group of people to know, and combats the isolation we often feel, and in addition teaches stretching and breathing techniques that are specifically helpful in dealing with stress. Some of us learn meditation.

Others work with one or another form of therapy. I myself am involved with re-evaluation co-counseling. Some of us find that at menopause our friendships with other women become close and important and very supportive. Whatever ways we have to deal with this stress will help produce home-brew estrogen.

An important part of the recipe is exercise. Exercise not only helps us feel better and function better but is specifically strengthening to our adrenal glands. Each of us needs to develop the kind of exercise program that is best for us. We need to think of exercise as part of our total life-change helping our bodies to produce estrogen.

My message about avoiding estrogen replacement, then, is not to suggest another magic potion. Our bodies do produce our own estrogen, but we need to give them the support and assistance that they need. Diet, stress reduction, and exercise will all help us in doing that.

WHY TAKE IT? YOU BE THE JUDGE

Promoters of estrogen would have us believe that menopause causes an estrogen deficiency disease that is mysterious and for which we need to take drugs. Estrogen in fact has been shown to be potentially helpful in reducing only two physical symptoms. Both of those are very noticeable if you have problems. So you can be the judge of whether even to consider taking estrogen. If you are not having problems, you do not need it.

Estrogen helps to reduce hot flashes and to relieve vaginal dryness. Neither hot flashes nor vaginal dryness will hurt you. They are not life-threatening. You can tell if you are having symptoms that are a problem to you. Too many doctors prescribe estrogen without ever knowing whether you have physical symptoms and whether you perceive them to be problems.

If you have hot flashes, you will know it! Some women experience them as sweats in the middle of the night. Others have a flush starting at the chest and radiating around the body. Some suddenly feel very stuffy and need air, and some feel prickles of perspiration suddenly. Hot flashes (or flushes) may or may not be severe. You may simply feel warm and observe the flush beginning, peaking, and receding. Or you may find your sleep disturbed or have severe flashes several times in an hour during the day.

If you perceive hot flashes to be a problem, there are a number of things you could try to relieve your symptoms without taking estrogen.

Ask your friends for hints on dealing with hot flashes.

> Wear layers! Summer or winter, so you always have something to take off and put back on when you get chilly from the flush. I find I can't wear synthetics anymore—it has to be cotton or wool.

> You know when you get a hot flash in the night and you throw the covers off because you're so hot and then you wake up later chilled? Stick one foot out of the covers instead! It will cool you down, and you won't get chills.

Some women find that taking vitamin E reduces the number and severity of hot flashes. Be cautious with the amount of vitamin E, as you would be with any medication. Many people probably take too much vitamin E; 600 IUs (international units) is probably the top safe level, and a very minimal amount of vitamin E (30 to 60 IUs) can produce good results for many women. Since so many women are diet conscious, they may have so little fat in the diet that they are actually deficient in vitamin E.

Here again we do need to rethink our concern about weight.

Since home-brew estrogen relies on the fatty tissue under the skin, and since a very restricted diet may result in deficiency in vitamin E, perhaps our health is better one size larger than we used to be.

The B vitamins also help in reducing hot flashes. In keeping with my basic theory that we need to let our bodies produce home-brew estrogen by reducing stress, we should remember that B vitamins are very helpful in dealing with stress. In fact, in health-food stores, a high-dose B-vitamin complex is often packaged with vitamin C as a "stress supplement."

Ginseng is a root that has been used medicinally in China for centuries. It has a normalizing effect on the pituitary. Some women find that it is more effective than vitamin E but some find that it is less effective. It is important to be careful and begin with very small amounts.

Reducing your sugar intake will very likely reduce the number and severity of your hot flashes. No research study has compared hot flashes among women who eat large amounts of food containing sugar and those who do not. Before recommending estrogen so routinely, doctors should encourage women to modify their diets.

Do not forget that alcohol is a very concentrated refined sugar. One woman said,

> After I had been off estrogen for a while, it got so that I had hot flashes only if I drank beer or wine or a drink, and I got hot flashes every time I had a drink.

Herbs are also potent drugs. People who are experts on herbs have some particular suggestions for reducing hot flashes. Among these are black cohosh and licorice root. I don't think licorice candy works! Proceed cautiously with herbs, as with any other potent drug. An herbalist or someone who works in an herb shop can often give helpful information. Magazines such as *Let's Live* and *Prevention* will sometimes have useful guides. Herbs, of course, will have more effect on our bodies the less polluted the body is with other substances such as sugar, caffeine, and alcohol.

VAGINAL DRYNESS

Low estrogen level is related to two changes in the vagina that can become problems. One, the walls of the vagina may become thinner and less elastic. Two, lubrication with sexual arousal takes longer to get started. Medically this condition is called "senile vaginal atrophy."

As men grow older it takes longer for them to get an erection and the penis is often less firm when erect. But doctors have not invented quite such a negative phrase for the natural changes in older men.

As with hot flashes, vaginal dryness is not life-threatening, and you will probably know if you have it. Although it takes sometimes a period of months before it is noticeable, women who have it are very aware of it. The walls of the vagina can become thinner instead of thick and corrugated, and the tissue may be less elastic. Intercourse can be extremely painful and could even cause bleeding if a woman has not made love for a long time. The pain from intercourse when the vagina is dry can last for several days. Any other kind of sexual activity leading to orgasm can be painful if the vagina contracts when it is not very elastic. Even if we do not have sexual activity, a dry vagina can be painful when we simply walk around.

The estrogen drugs do help the walls of the vagina become thicker and less likely to bleed or cause pain. But at what cost? We have learned from the story of DES (diethylstilbestrol) that estrogen drugs can have delayed consequences. There is a Premarin cream that is inserted into the vagina. It had been thought to be less hazardous than taking estrogen by mouth, but recent research shows that vaginal applications of drugs are assimilated into the general system even faster than oral drugs. If sexual changes are the only problem you are experiencing, and if you choose to use estrogen, do consider estrogen cream rather than estrogen by mouth. But do not be fooled that it will not be absorbed into your body.

A forty-year-old woman reported,

> I had not taken estrogen cream or estrogen by mouth for two years. When I began to use estrogen cream twice a week, I noticed changes immediately. After the first time I inserted it, my breasts became slightly firmer in texture. I liked it, but I wonder where else the hormones are going and what they will do to me.

Researchers and doctors are concerned about the effects of estrogen cream on the bladder and kidney system.

If you are noticing sexual problems and want to try an alternative to taking estrogen, we will again discuss a variety of things. Many women notice that vitamin E and ginseng are helpful. Ginseng in fact has the reputation, perhaps stretched, of being an aphrodisiac. Vitamin E oil is soothing to the tissue in your vulva and has specific properties similar to estrogen. In addition, the B vitamins and zinc are frequently recommended to improve sexual functioning. One way to know if you have a zinc deficiency is to notice whether you have white spots on your fingernails. These apparently indicate a deficiency in zinc.

Another kind of change you may notice in your vagina is that the acid balance, or pH balance, changes. The norm during our adult years is to have a rather acid vagina. There are a number of organisms, such as yeast, which normally live in the vagina. If the pH of the vagina becomes less acid, then those bacteria can multiply and cause irritation or infection. After menopause the pH may become less acid. In addition, eating sugar causes the pH to be less acid and the sugar can cause the yeast to grow and multiply. Taking estrogen drugs, though, also affects the pH and may trigger a growth of yeast. If your vagina has more yeast or a less acid environment than usual, it can feel very easily irritated and intercourse can be painful.

Teresa, thirty-two, described it this way.

Since my ovaries were taken out I sometimes get what I think is going to be a yeast infection but it never gets that bad. It is a little bit of white discharge, it smells sweet and yeasty, and it makes my vulva sore. After a while it goes away. I'm positive that I get it every time I go on a cookie binge.

Douching with yogurt can help to reestablish a good vaginal pH. Vinegar or other douche products are too harsh for older women's vaginas, and the yogurt helps to regulate the growth of yeast. If you do use yogurt, you can spoon it in and hold it in with a tampon or put it in before you go to bed so you will lie down for a while. Use the freshest yogurt you can find, so the culture will be live.

Two articles claim evidence from animal studies that THC (tetrahydrocannabinol), the active ingredient in marijuana, may have an estrogen-like effect on women's sexual organs.

Another alternative to estrogen replacement is again exercise. Here I mean exercise of our sexual organs. There is a great deal of evidence that if we remain sexually active, we will be exercising more and are less likely to have as severe problems with vaginal lubrication.

For most of us the more often we are sexually aroused, the more quickly we become lubricated. In addition, we need to retrain our sexual partners to go slower . . . to accommodate our longer arousal time. If we are relating to men, many of them also have a slower arousal time during the middle age.

We need to help ourselves take pleasure in all kinds of touching and caressing and pleasurable activities. These activities will not only help us be more relaxed and enjoy sex more, but will also have a specific effect on our genital organs.

Many of us do not have sexual partners with whom we can explore new ways of sexual functioning. Masturbation is great physical therapy. If we can put aside some time that is just for us, if we can get some oil, some apricot-kernel oil, or some vitamin E oil, and explore our bodies and recover some of the sensuality all by ourselves, then we will be helping our bodies to keep on functioning well sexually.

OSTEOPOROSIS

I have been saying "You be the judge" as to whether you need to take estrogen. If vaginal changes or hot flashes are a problem, you will know it. The one condition for which estrogen has been promoted that we may not be able to judge ourselves is osteoporosis. Osteoporosis is the thinning of the bones from a loss of calcium.

Osteoporosis is a serious problem, and we should think about ways to prevent it. It is not the reduced bone mass itself that is a problem, but the possibility of fracture. You know how worried we get about older women who fall, because they are so likely to break a bone. Robert Heaney reported in the national conference on menopause and aging in 1971 that

> approximately 25 percent of all white women over age 60 have spinal compression fractures due to osteoporosis, and the risk of hip fracture is at least 20 percent by age 90. . . . This fracture is perhaps the most sinister manifestation of osteoporosis, as 1/6 of all hip fracture patients died within three months of injury.

Clear information on the relationship of osteoporosis and estrogen replacement therapy continues to be unavailable. One expert called osteoporosis a "disease of theories" when it comes to explaining the precise relationship between ovarian function and bone metabolism. Estrogens if given at menopause can retard bone loss, but if the estrogens are discontinued the bone loss can accelerate. This is very significant for women having premature menopause. It means that if a woman begins to take estrogen, she must continue to take it indefinitely or the potentially beneficial effects of the estrogen are eliminated.

A reassuring study about estrogen and osteoporosis has been

criticized medically. It is the study by Lila Nachtigall, and it showed fewer hip fractures in the group of women who were receiving estrogen. One problem with the study is that the women were in a hospital for chronic disease. Their exercise level was certainly very low, and their diet may have been quite deficient. They were not taking calcium supplements or extra vitamins. The study is of women in the poorest health. You and I can take more steps to prevent osteoporosis than they did.

Calcium supplements have been shown to delay bone loss and large doses of 1 to 1.5 grams per day are generally recommended for post-menopausal women. One expert recommends a single late evening dose. Although the research is mixed, vitamin D supplements may also be recommended to raise the calcium metabolism.

Calcium supplements have additional benefits. Calcium is an effective mild tranquilizer, and many people find that it helps them to sleep. A glass of warm milk before bedtime has been used for years as a gentle sleeping potion.

Exercise also is important for preventing osteoporosis. Some experts believe exercise can help prevent osteoporosis and slow its progression.

As we help our bodies by supplying calcium, we need to watch our intake of phosphorus and magnesium. The "normal American diet" is very high in phosphorus, and that prevents the absorption of calcium. A semivegetarian diet low in meat and high in eggs and milk is probably best for keeping calcium high and phosphorus low. The proportions recommended are that the amount of calcium we ingest should be double the amount of magnesium and at least equal to that of phosphorus. It is also important to take sufficient vitamin D, which we can get from sunshine or vitamin D–enriched milk. We are likely to find we have four or five times the amount of phosphorus as calcium each day.

Evidence from many different studies suggests that osteoporosis is related far more to general health than to estrogen. In cultures where women remain physically active longer than men, it is men who get osteoporosis earlier than women.

A sidelight of following my prescription for home-brew estrogen could be an improvement in your dental health. It has been noticed that women who are postmenopausal sometimes have gum problems that can lead to severe tooth decay. Vigorous exercise, a diet with fewer refined foods, and supplements such as vitamin C can probably arrest these changes.

OTHER EFFECTS

Medical researchers have not documented some of the other changes women notice when they take estrogen. Some women notice a feeling of well-being. It could be that the drugs cause an elevation in blood sugar, thus promoting a temporary euphoria.

Another change reported by some women is that their skin seems to improve when they take estrogen. The research by the Feminist Women's Health Centers provides a possible explanation for that.

> The body's real estrogen is known to be important for healthy skin and mucous membranes inside and outside the body. Estrogen is believed to cause the cells to retain water, to increase sugar and fat in the blood, and to regulate calcium storage in the bones. Real estrogens maintain the skin's health by stimulating the skin cells. Estrogen-like drugs create the illusion of healthier, younger skin by making it retain more water which in turn temporarily smoothes out wrinkles.

DON'T TAKE ESTROGEN, TAKE CHARGE

Making a decision about taking estrogen is very difficult for most of us. We are alternately frightened by reports that give us the feeling we will die immediately on ingesting a single pill and by reports that reassure us that no harm can come from taking estrogen. Each of us must do our own risk-assessment.

Lila Nachtigall has made the statement that estrogen does not cause cancer. That statement is based on the fact that no researcher can say without a doubt that estrogen causes cancer. What researchers can say is that if you look at many, many women, the women who take estrogen tend to have certain problems more frequently than women who do not. No statistician can infer causation from correlation. That is drilled into any elementary statistics student.

But your personal concern is your own risk. On the one hand you will probably not get cancer if you take estrogen. Most women who take estrogen do not get cancer. Most women who take estrogen do not get gallbladder disease. The problem is that if you take estrogen, you have a higher risk of those illnesses. You may be able to be more specific about your own personal risks. Have you had gallbladder disease? Or has a family member had gallbladder disease? Has your mother had an estrogen-related cancer? Have you had any effects from birth control pills? Those are questions that should be considered when you are calculating your own personal risk factor.

The figures about osteoporosis include all women. If you are from northern European background and are fairly small in stature, you have a higher risk of osteoporosis than if you are a Mediterranean or third-world person. If you smoke cigarettes you have a higher risk. So in considering your personal risk of osteoporosis compared to your personal risk of problems with estrogens, you must consider your unique body and background. Also, remember that taking estrogens and then stopping can increase the risk of osteoporosis.

Taking progestin is recommended to reduce the risks of taking estrogen, and it is said that progestins are safe. That statement can be made today because thorough research on the effects of estrogens and progestins has not been done. It is true that no research shows a hazard associated with progestin, but no research truly shows that it is safe.

The other part of taking charge in your own risk-assessment is deciding which risks you can act to reduce. If you take estrogen, we know of little now that you can do to reduce the risk of cancer. If you do not take estrogen, there are a number of things you can do to reduce the risk of osteoporosis. You can take calcium supplements, and you can exercise.

When researchers and policy analysts talk about the cost-benefit ratios of a plan of taking estrogen or not, they are speaking of women in the aggregate, or large groups of women. You and I can take charge of our own bodies. We can take steps to reduce our risks of osteoporosis, and we can take steps to reduce the hot flashes or vaginal dryness we may experience.

Each of us must make our own decision. We do not live in a world where taking good care of ourselves is easy. For some of us my prescription for home-brew estrogen may appear impossible. You may continue to take estrogen, and you probably will not have a major trauma from it. The problem is, you don't know.

DETOX

What if you are taking estrogen and want to reduce it? Here I will use an analogy from my work in the drug-abuse field. Estrogen is a dangerous drug to which we become habituated. Just as with any other drug it is very difficult to go "cold turkey," to stop suddenly. If you can do it, fine. Prepare for some withdrawal symptoms like increased hot flashes and wait it out.

You may prefer to embark on a gradual detoxification program. Check to see what dose of estrogen you are taking. Many women take .6 milligrams, and the lowest dosage is .035 milligrams. Ask your doctor for a prescription for the dosage a step lower than the one you have now. Your doctor may be able to assist you in your detox program, by recommending a schedule of withdrawal. But your doctor may be no help at all and may warn you of dire results if you reduce your dose of estrogen.

I recommend that women consider starting their own detox program, even without a doctor's support. Of course, you should listen very carefully to the reasons the doctor gives and question very thoroughly whether there is some condition specific to you that makes taking estrogen crucial.

Rosetta Reitz, having traveled the country twice speaking with women, and having received large amounts of correspondence, is also very much aware of the need for detox. In a telephone interview she said,

> I have found lots of women who have been frightened and intimidated by doctors who suddenly take them off estrogen. They want to learn how to get off estrogen if they can, but are given no support. . . . Many have become addicted to estrogen. I have developed a detox pattern that goes like this. The first month, don't take the pill the eleventh day. The second month, omit the seventh and fourteenth day.

The third month, eliminate three pills, evenly spaced. And so on until gradually you eliminate the estrogen. At the same time, you need to build your body through nutrition and exercise.

Here is the experience of Sylvia, whose ovaries were removed when she was thirty-two and who decided after a year and a half to go off estrogen:

> The detox pattern that I followed was to switch to the lowest dosage by alternating higher and lower doses daily for a couple of weeks and then using all the lower dose. For myself I found that the three-weeks-on, one-week-off cycle of taking estrogen was terrible. I always got bad hot flashes after I stopped it and when I started it again. I began to take it every other day without the pause for one week.

Doctors prescribe taking estrogen for three weeks and off for one week so that women will "bleed" and the uterine lining will not build up. That is not a problem for a woman who has had a hysterectomy.

Sylvia continues,

> Switching to every-other-day estrogen evened out my symptoms a lot. Then I found I was forgetting to take it sometimes. Two days would go by, then I'd take one. Gradually I forgot more and more. There came a time when I realized I had not taken any for over a week. For six months or so I still had occasional hot flashes, especially if I drank alcohol. I would take extra vitamin B if I ever did drink alcohol and that seemed to help.

That kind of gradual withdrawal seems to make sense. But as with whether to take estrogen at all, you should be the judge. If you embark on a withdrawal program and at the same time follow my prescription for home-brew estrogen, you will undoubtedly feel much better. We truly do not need to be captives of a tiny dangerous pill.

Chapter Ten

HEALTH and HEALING

For every woman a hysterectomy has its own unique meaning. Every woman grows from a hysterectomy experience. The operation may inspire you to take much better care of yourself physically. It could cause you to do some needed emotional work. The operation may stimulate you to explore some otherwise hidden feelings about yourself. It might trigger greater assertiveness in your encounters with the medical profession. It may become the focus of political action. Even a negative experience holds the potential for growth.

Addie, who is forty, reflects on the meaning of her hysterectomy.

It's been five years now. In retrospect, it was a bad experience. I didn't do the checking and investigating I might have done, and I think my hysterectomy maybe could have been avoided. But since then I am far less self-critical than I used to be. If I have a problem, I don't blame it on myself as much as I used to. I think at the time of the hysterectomy I hit bottom, and although it's a terrible cost, I think I'm getting better now.

Grace was forty-two when she had a hysterectomy. That experience caused her to reflect on her priorities and her life.

It's different if you have cancer. Then the hysterectomy seems trivial and you suddenly rearrange all your priorities. I found like every other cancer patient I've talked to, that every day seems very precious to me now. I miss my uterus, but I love the rest of my body more than I ever did before.

Sharon's hysterectomy had an impact on her marriage.

I once read an article by Hugh Drummond in *Mother Jones* magazine about marriage. It said sometimes the need for women to be subordinate to men in marriage even causes the women to become seriously ill. I think that is what happened to me. As I look back, I got sick after a terribly stressful time for my husband. He has said many times he could never recover from my hysterectomy, and now he says the hysterectomy has cost him a marriage. I feel terribly hurt, but I think I'm going to be better off on my own. So I guess maybe the meaning of the hysterectomy for me is in forcing me to deal with our relationship.

Sylvia sees her hysterectomy as an important symbol of a change in her life.

The whole thing means I can't get pregnant anymore and for me that means everything. I haven't had any trouble with the operation, and I feel like I'm entering a whole new time of my life.

HELP IN HEALING

The most important help you can give a woman you care about in healing from a hysterectomy is to think well about her. That does not mean think for her, and it does not mean you tell her all your thoughts. It means you should think about her strengths and how you can remind her of her strengths if she is feeling weak. It means you think about her "blind spots" and as subtly as you possibly can, provide new visions in those areas. It means you listen extremely well and watch for cues of feelings to be expressed. It means you put aside your own feelings about the topic or about her problems and talk with someone else about your own feelings. Your job is to be there for her.

As you think well about the woman you care about, your actions will be in three major areas:

1. *Good listening*

More than anything else, your friend needs a good listener. She needs you to look interested, even if you have heard her talk about it before. She needs you to bite your tongue if you were about to jump in and tell your own story or other stories you have heard. During this time you should try to think three times before saying anything. Most of us have very little experience in talking to a good listener. Simply talking to a good listener often helps a woman solve her own problems. After all, she has all the information about her own body and her own experience.

You need to be a very permissive listener. You need to give her permission to express unacceptable feelings. They are all part of her experience, and she needs to have the safety to express them.

If you see she is close to tears, figure out a way to help her cry. Sometimes if you see her eyes filling, you can say, "Would you like a hug?" or "It's fine to cry." If her voice rises in anger, now is not the time to argue whether her position is rational or not.

Encourage her to yell and beat a pillow, and she will be able to think more clearly later.

If you have any experience with communication skills training or parent effectiveness training, here is where to use the techniques of active listening. As an active listener you reflect back to her your best judgment of what she is saying. That will assist her to continue to clarify her own thinking.

As you listen, note the areas she slides over. They may be topics truly of little concern, or they may be overwhelming to her. Then later figure out a way to gently introduce the topic. For example you might say, "Many women have feelings about not being able to have more children, even if they have already had their family." Or you might say, "I just realized you haven't been in a hospital except ages ago when your children were born. What's that going to be like for you?"

2. Provide information appropriately

You have a different perspective on the hysterectomy experience than she does, so you may be able to seek and provide information that could be helpful to her. But we have all had the experience of rushing up to someone with new, exciting information and finding them unreceptive. You need to plan the most effective way to provide information for her.

Information may be from written material, or it may be about local support groups she could find helpful, organized around such subjects as infertility, menopause, or hysterectomy itself. You may be able to locate a good doctor to give her a second opinion, and perhaps that would ensure her taking that very crucial step.

If your friend has not had a hysterectomy, probably the most important information you can provide is that first, she has a right to a second opinion, and second, there may be other options besides hysterectomy. You as her friend may be able to investigate some of the options, although of course you cannot push her into anything she is not ready to do. Many women truly want someone to give them permission and information to support their saying no to the gynecologist and not having a hysterectomy. You may be able to provide that support for your friend.

3. *Be with her*

Just as with a second opinion it is hard to underestimate the significance of accompanying a woman to a doctor visit. The changes are very subtle, but with you there your friend will be a different person. She will be able to think more clearly because you are there silently reminding her of the strong woman she is outside the doctor's office. It is especially important for women to accompany other women.

As her advocate you can ask the doctor questions you think she may have but has not yet asked. You can help her ahead of time to make a list of questions for the doctor, and you can talk with her after the visit and encourage her to telephone the doctor with any further questions.

It can also be very helpful for you to go with her as she checks into the hospital. Once she returns home, there will be many ways you can be specifically helpful to her in running her household.

Be alert also to a woman's need to be alone. Many women are so accustomed to tuning in to the needs of others that it is very hard for them to relax when other people are around. It may be that you can devote your energies most effectively after surgery to assisting in her household behind the scenes. Telephone calls in the hospital may for some women be more helpful than a visit in person.

4. *Notes for men*

For men who are concerned about a woman having a hysterectomy, all of the above suggestions are relevant. In addition, you need to be especially careful to deal with your feelings about her hysterectomy somewhere else. In most relationships between men and women the woman provides much of the emotional support for the man. In a hysterectomy situation you will need emotional support to deal with feelings about her experience. If you talk about them very much with her, your feelings will come in as requests for help. It is not appropriate for her to provide help for you. She needs to do her own healing, and you should talk with others about your feelings. You may find you can locate a counselor and arrange a short-term program of sessions, or you may find a friend who can listen to you talk. When you talk with the woman who has had the hysterectomy, you should be able to put aside your own feelings and truly be there for her.

Much of your uncertainty will originate in your need for information. Read this book and others to find some answers to your questions, and do not hesitate to ask for professional advice. A woman's doctor should be willing to answer your questions as well as hers. You need to know she will heal, that she is resilient and strong. You need to keep telling her you know she is resilient and strong. She will be unable to do some of her everyday activities for a period of days or weeks or months. She will need extra help with household responsibilities. And she may be told not to drive or to climb stairs or to lift.

She will heal sexually, and you do not need to worry that you might injure her after the doctor says sex is all right. Take extra care to remember all the ways to make love. All the touching and kissing and stroking will help your relationship and will help her heal. Now may be a time to go back and explore some of the ways of making love in addition to intercourse, since intercourse may be delayed for several weeks.

Ralph is the husband of a woman who had a hysterectomy at forty-five.

> It upset me more than I ever thought it would to see her in the hospital. All of a sudden I worried that she might die. I wish I could have talked about it with someone, like my minister, because it really took awhile for me to get over the shock of seeing her in the hospital after the operation.

Jim made a special point of being extra supportive to his wife when she had a hysterectomy.

> I was her main cheering squad. I went with her to the doctor sometimes and whenever she felt low I kept telling her I

knew she could do it and she would be fine. She is a dynamite lady, and she came through with flying colors. What help could I have used? Oh, nothing, it wasn't a problem for me.

Women are very specific about what they want from their friends and lovers. They will describe what has been useful for them, what help they could have done without, and what they would have liked more of.

My best support was the assistant minister in my church. We were in a class she was teaching about sexuality and it turned out she was going to have a hysterectomy herself. We started talking and it was a big help for me. She listened to me and I felt she did not confuse me with her. I felt like her experience as a minister helped, but she said I was helpful to her too. I think it was just good to have someone to talk to.

As I think back on it, different people did for me the things they do best. One friend works in a library, and she got lots of information for me. She's the one who found out about the infertility support group too. There was something about the way she told me about them, that I could take the information or not. I didn't feel pressured. Then my neighbor took my children while I was in the hospital and cooked extra food. My husband was really taking care of the house, but behind the scenes she helped a lot. He never could have done it without her and I would have worried if she hadn't been helping. My sister turned out to be the best one to talk to. She hasn't had a hysterectomy but I know she loves me no matter what I do or say. I had a couple late-night conversations with her before my operation and once or twice since where I really let my hair down. What I love about talking to her is I don't feel she really remembers what I say when I'm upset. My husband was the one who went along with me to the hospital and came the most to visit me. I felt very close to him in those times, like he was holding my hand as I went near dying and came back again. Once in a while I felt like he was afraid, but he didn't let on to me.

I think it was different for me because I'm a lesbian. I have a whole group of friends and acquaintances who try very hard to support me and other women. My lover was incredibly wonderful. She was always gentle and tender with me and somehow I got the feeling she was lending me some of her strength. My friends seemed to have the right balance of taking it all very seriously but letting me joke about it too. We had a good-bye party for my womb before I went to the hospital. I said what I liked about it and why I would miss it and why I was glad it was going, and they all said what they liked about me and why they knew I would come out strong. Everyone remembers that night as one of the best times we've ever had.

Women generally have bad experiences because a well-meaning other person puts his or her own feelings ahead of thinking about the woman. Many of the stories of bad experiences describe doctors' behavior, but friends can be unthinking also.

I got absolutely no support from my doctor about anything except drugs for the pain. I wanted to think about whether the hysterectomy even made sense or what kinds of changes would happen, but I felt I was bothering him if I ever said anything.

I tried and tried to ask questions but maybe I couldn't ask them well enough, but the doctors kept not answering my questions. It was only one intern in the hospital who took the time to explain a lot to me.

My doctor explained a lot but she still wasn't a source of the emotional support I needed.

This whole hysterectomy experience almost cost me one friendship. My friend kept bringing me more and more horror stories of awful things that had happened to other women when they had hysterectomies. Maybe she was doing it for my own good, but I really couldn't listen to all that.

Since I was only in my twenties and hadn't had children, whenever I said I was going to have a hysterectomy other people's faces would take on this look of terrible pity. I couldn't stand it. My friends would stop talking about babies when I came into the room. I felt like all of a sudden I was a different person and they had to tiptoe around me. I really wanted them to just go on and be normal.

With one of my friends in particular I felt like I was her "cause." She was very upset about unnecessary hysterectomy, and I felt she was trying hard to talk me out of it. That's okay, but she wasn't giving me any answers or any support for the problems I was having.

Before my operation all my friends were talking about how great they felt after, how they never had any trouble. Since I haven't recovered too fast and I've been feeling pretty low, I have trouble being around them. It seems like they're telling me I'm not coping as well as they did.

As women look back on the support and information they received, they often speak of wishing their friends had given them more information or more support for expressing feelings.

It wasn't until later I found out one of my friends knows about adoption. If she had told me some of the things before my surgery, I would have been able to make plans or fantasies about adoption while I was thinking about hysterectomy.

I'm a very rational person and what I wanted more from my friends was for them to let me be irrational. Everyone knew

I could cope and could think well about things, but I wanted to be able to be just a little girl again.

As I look back on it, I think I was looking for someone to tell me not to have the hysterectomy. Everyone was trying so hard not to influence me but I think if someone had firmly said you don't have to do this now I would have waited.

ANALYSIS INTO ACTION

Hysterectomy is not just a personal issue. It is a reflection of problems in society and in the health system, and it is a symptom of deeper hurts than any one individual can experience. We must not only help one another as individuals to cope with hysterectomy, but we must also work together to change the entire framework of health care and women's experience.

As individuals we must think of ourselves first. We must provide ourselves the nurturing and support we need. This is an individual action, yet it contradicts such heavy social conditioning that it represents social change as well. If all women stopped compulsively nurturing others and compulsively putting themselves last, we would see some major social changes. Nurturing is wonderful and important, and we must not lose our skills at nurturing others. But for almost all women, to put ourselves first is a powerful political statement.

For many of us enormous anger is connected with hysterectomy, whether it is our hysterectomy or that of someone close to us. We must care for one another so we can heal from the anger. We must allow one another opportunities to rage so the anger is not turned inward. But then we must turn the anger into action. We must work together to end abuse of all women.

If you have had a bad experience with hysterectomy, you are not alone. Your experience is similar to that of thousands of women across the country. You can take actions to support those women and also to prevent future experiences such as yours.

If you have had a good experience with hysterectomy, your experience is also not unique. Thousands of women have very good experiences with hysterectomy. We need to share those triumphs, because they are testaments to the enormous vitality and resilience of women.

Any action you take will be crucial. Here are some suggestions of what other women have done.

1. *Talk with people*

Share your experiences. Especially as you find the ways to tell your experience without expecting your listener to take the same path you did, your sharing your story with other women will be very helpful. Every woman you talk with will feel less isolated. Every woman who feels less isolated will act more powerfully. Every woman who acts more powerfully changes, however minutely, the social experience of women today.

2. *Be a friend*

Offer to go with friends to doctor visits. Look up information and make it available to your friends. Strongly encourage your friends to get second opinions for any surgery. Follow all of the suggestions I listed above on thinking well about your friends.

3. *Take appropriate actions for yourself*

File a lawsuit if that is appropriate. File a complaint if you have had poor care in a health setting. As individual lawsuits and complaints become part of a larger picture they help set the scene for policy changes.

4. *Organize a group*

You could put a notice in a local women's center and a local church, as I did in Boston, and collect a small group of women to meet in your home once or twice. Or you could form an organization to provide counseling and advocacy for women experiencing hysterectomy, as Leslie Hanover in Los Angeles did when she formed the group Womb 'n Awareness. The group enrolls members, provides a newsletter, public lectures, and a medical and psychological referral service. Groups are helpful for the women who participate, and the existence of the group also changes the climate of hush and mystery surrounding hysterectomy.

5. *Teach a class*

You may have the opportunity to organize a class in your community or your workplace. Many public libraries and clinics have regular classes, and you could offer to teach one on hysterectomy. You may be able to see that a class about hysterectomy is provided for social workers or for nurses or for counselors, if one of those is your profession.

6. *Publicize local issues*

If you have had a bad experience or a good experience, contact local women's groups, women's centers, and women's clinics. They often have referral networks, and your information will be very valuable. Write letters to the editor of your newspaper, commenting on articles that reveal or cover up local problems you may be aware of.

7. *Plug into advocacy networks*

Hysterectomy is only part of the whole picture of health care and women's experience. The way hysterectomy is abused is related to other issues. Become familiar with local groups organizing around the issues of health care for women, health care for poor people, environmental health issues, abortion rights, and the rights of minority groups. We must assume all our struggles are linked and act on that assumption.

8. *Work for social change*

The large number of unnecessary hysterectomies, the poor support many women receive in the hysterectomy experience, and the lack of options for treatment of problems women have, all are results of a society in which women and minority group members are in a relatively powerless position and in which the health system is profit-oriented. Change in any area of society will at some level influence women's experience with the health system, so any social-change work you do will have an impact on the hysterectomy experience.

Women today are incredibly resourceful, nurturing, strong, and competent. We do have a major problem with unnecessary hysterectomies. But we are doing something about that problem. Every woman who has talked with me or with someone else is part of the solution of the problem.

Appendix I:

ALTERNATIVE HEALING METHODS

Until one hundred years ago doctors practicing what we know as modern medicine were a small sect competing with other forms of healing. Today many other kinds of healing are again becoming increasingly visible. Under the label of the holistic health movement we find professional healers and many different approaches to self-care.

Among professional healers there are many chiropractors who will assist a person in a general plan for health in addition to working on the person's back or neck. Naturopaths have a specific theory that is opposite to allopathic medicine; they prescribe tiny doses of substances that simulate an illness, as opposed to the allopathic approach of strong medicines that contradict the illness. The training of osteopaths is similar to that of regular doctors but has some additional holistic elements. Christian Science practitioners have a long history of healing without the use of medicines.

Most common under the holistic health umbrella are healers

who combine a number of approaches and methods. They may come from a wide variety of training and backgrounds. An alternative healer may be trained as a doctor or a nurse, a chiropractor or an herbalist, a psychotherapist or an acupuncturist. Finding an alternative healer is often very difficult. Because of their (probably realistic) fear of harassment by the medical establishment, many alternative healers are not very visible. The best way to find an alternative healer who will work well with you is to shop and ask around. Health food stores can be good places to ask, and people you know may know of alternative healers.

We have been taught to be very suspicious of alternative healers and to call them "quacks." The public image of alternative healers as quacks has been deliberately promoted by the medical doctors. Although there are certainly unethical practitioners and ineffective treatments in the holistic area, there are just as certainly unethical medical practitioners and ineffective medical treatment. If a healer or a method shows a success rate, that person must have part of the answer to the question of how to treat some people or some problems.

Books and magazines can also be excellent sources of information about alternative methods of healing. Reading about a method of treatment is very different from working with a practitioner who will make a specific proposal for your healing, but it is an excellent way to begin to shop around. Health food stores sell books that take a wide variety of approaches to healing, and many general bookstores have a large health section. It can be very confusing, since each method may claim to have the entire answer, but as you use your own good sense you will elicit the information most helpful to you.

An excellent overview of self-care and a review of other books is Donald B. Ardell's *High Level Wellness*. A good basic resource is Mark Bricklin's *The Practical Encyclopedia of Natural Healing*. Although the book is shamefully weak in the area of women's problems, it does have basic information about many approaches to healing. A forthcoming book that will be extremely valuable is by Kay Weiss, to be published by Reston Publishing Company and tentatively titled *Women's Medicine: Alternative Treatments.*

As you ask around you will find women have obtained assistance from a wide variety of sources.

Jonell: I am a librarian, so I can see practically every book that comes out. But I found my library did not have very many books about alternative medicine. I was chatting with some of the regular patrons and got turned on to the book selection in my local health food store. I have ordered some of the best books for our library, so now they are available to more people.

Patricia: I started going to a chiropractor because I hurt my back. I noticed that he had little pots of vitamins that he sold and found out that he did nutritional analysis and suggested special vitamins for particular problems. I have started going to him when I have other problems not just with my back, and I find it is much better than my doctor. If I have a true infection, he will send me to the doctor for a culture or blood test and antibiotics, but he uses acupuncture, massage, vitamins, and I don't know what else. He says his approach is like the touch-for-health system.

Sylvia: The nutritionist I go to is not like any nutritionist I ever heard of. Some people say she is psychic, she says she uses many different theories and has studied with many different people. She herself was healed by Dr. Henry Bieler, who wrote the book *Food Is Your Best Medicine.* I find the book all right, but seeing her is much better for me. She tells me specifically what foods I can eat and what foods I can't digest well, and at different times in my life, she has given me very different diet plans. It was freaky the first time I saw her, because she gave a different analysis for every person in the group. And she told me to avoid certain foods that I know I am very allergic to.

Sharon:

Karen:

She didn't tell anyone else in the group to avoid those foods. Staying on her diet is very hard work, though. I heard about her from people in my food co-op who had gone to her.

I couldn't believe it. Here I was going to the Kaiser health plan and I started talking to my doctor and found out he worked part-time at the holistic health center. He's a regular M.D., but he gave me more ideas about diet and exercise and he also gave me referrals to several different people.

I found out about my doctor at a workshop she did which a friend of mine had attended. She is a highly trained medical doctor, and has studied Eastern philosophy intensively. Her work is an integration of Eastern philosophy and Western medicine. I have been very happy going to her.

Just as regular medicine does not have the total answer to the question of how to heal us, neither does any one alternative method. Each of us needs to choose our own combination of approaches, since each of us has different needs and different available resources. These are some of the approaches that people have used in healing.

EXERCISE

Exercise is probably one of the most fundamental steps we can take to make ourselves healthier. Any increase in the amount of exercise we have will improve our general health, and some particular exercises can help with particular problems. Walking, swimming, and active sports are exercises that will improve circulation, breathing, and flexibility. Sources of information about specific exercise programs for you could be a chiropractor, a physical therapist, or a skillful instructor of swimming, dancing, or aerobic exercise. You might find that a program of exercise for older people could be very helpful as a gentle healing program, even if you are not old.

Yoga is a form of exercise that has specific healing properties. There are many excellent instructors and centers that teach yoga exercise. Yoga in general improves breathing, circulation, and flexibility, and some positions have a particular healing effect on certain organs. You will find many good books on yoga, including the classic ones by Hittleman, such as *Be Young with Yoga*. The Bricklin *Encyclopedia of Natural Healing* has a good section on yoga positions for specific ailments.

NUTRITION

A second fundamental way to improve our health is to improve our nutrition. Most of us can benefit from a basic program of improved diet, using any of the books or resources that teach us about the harmful effects of refined sugars, alcohol, and stimulants. Many doctors and other healers believe that vitamin and mineral supplements are helpful for everyone to counteract the depleted nutritive properties of the foods we eat. Some people also recommend specific vitamins or mineral supplements for specific problems. *Prevention* magazine is a good source of information on supplements as well as on other health issues. My favorite books on menopause and estrogen, the Seamans' *Women and the Crisis in Sex Hormones* and Rosetta Reitz's *Menopause: A Positive Approach,* both include detailed information on supplements that can be helpful to women.

Herbal medicines are also vitamin supplements, but must be considered potent medicines and approached very cautiously. A recent encyclopedia-style book of herbs is *The Rodale Herb Book,* edited by William Hylton.

Another approach to nutritional treatment involves cleansing or fasting. Individuals sometimes find that periodic fasting for twenty-four hours or more, or a juice fast, or a specific cleansing involving enemas and fasting are very helpful in general well-being. Healers sometimes propose specific plans of modified fasting for longer periods of time, involving avoiding foods the body cannot handle well in order to promote healing. A good source of information on diet and cleansing fasting is the work of Paavo Airola.

TREATMENTS INVOLVING THE MIND

Many people find that meditation is very helpful in dealing with the stress in everyday life. Some people practice transcendental meditation, others develop their own meditation strategy. For people with health problems meditation frequently has a definite healing effect.

A more specific way of working on health problems is the method of visualization. Visualization involves a guided meditation process. Therapists can lead you in visualization, or you can work on visualization by yourself. Books such as *The Well-Body Book* by Hal Bennett and Michael Samuels have helpful instructions for your own visualization. Visualization can involve constructing a picture of your body as healthy, it can involve imaging healing going to your hurt parts, such as the hurt parts being washed with water or filled with light, and it can involve visualizing your whole body covered with healing light or with a particular color.

MASSAGE

Massage can be an extremely relaxing and soothing method of dealing with everyday life stresses. Some people find a good person and arrange for a massage regularly every month, for the healing properties of the massage.

Some specific healing methods involve massage of particular points. Acupressure is based on the acupuncture points of Chinese medicine. It involves massage or pressure on certain points that are related to particular body parts. Acupressure can be used as a specific treatment for an ailment, and it also can be a general toning massage. Acupressure massage sometimes is called Shiatsu.

Reflexology, or zone therapy, is also a form of massage using particular points to stimulate or heal particular organs. The work of Mildred Carter, including one book on foot-reflexology and one on hand-reflexology, can be very helpful. The theory is that the foot or the hand are a map of the body parts and massage of a particular point can heal the ailing part.

The *Touch for Health* system developed by John Thie is a method combining some acupressure theory and some chiropractic technique. Touch-for-health classes or workshops are taught in some communities, and the methods can be used to identify ailments and also to identify foods or medicines that the body can or cannot handle. Many chiropractors use touch-for-health methods, as well as acupressure and acupuncture treatments.

As you investigate options in healing remember that our bodies, minds, and spirits are very complex and there are many ways to interpret and understand the relationships between them. Each approach to healing has part of the picture, and we can learn important information from each. If it seems confusing in that all the approaches are conflicting and competing, remember to contrast them with the traditional practice of medicine. Frequently regular medicine appears by far the most narrow and restricted approach to healing. Tune in to what is going on for your body, and what is best for you, and you will adopt a good approach.

Self-healing is a long process and requires attention, energy, and care. For many of us it is far easier to stay with regular medicine. Self-healing requires effort in choosing a practitioner or a method, generally requires more attention to nutrition, and often requires other life-style changes.

If you do decide to embark on self-healing, get support for yourself. Tell your friends what you are doing and ask specifically for their help. You may find you become discouraged and backslide. Don't be self-critical if that happens, but pick up and start again. The effects of self-healing will last the rest of your life.

Marian: Here I am in a small city in the Midwest. I don't have access to all these alternative healers I hear people on the coasts talk about. I'm lucky to get a doctor who is decent to me. I'm trying to improve my health by things I read, but when it comes to my endometriosis, I'm letting the doctor help me.

Clara: I'm putting out a lot of energy right now on healing, and it's taking enormous amounts of time and some money. I know I can do this only because I'm a student and on vacation and I don't have children. It seems like it would be overwhelming if I had more pressures in my life.

Nancy: The very first steps in my self-help progress paid off. The first things the nutritionist said to do were to stop coffee and sugar, and there was something about the confidence she inspired in me that made me go right home and do it immediately. I have felt better ever since and it really inspires me to keep on. Also, I started exercising and that right now really keeps itself going.

Appendix II:

THE PSYCHOLOGICAL RESEARCH on HYSTERECTOMY

How will a woman feel after a hysterectomy? What psychological effects might there be? That is a hard question to answer by looking at the published research. Some studies, asking short questions ("Have you been happy since your hysterectomy?"), find that women generally say they are fine. Other studies, doing in-depth interviews, find that hysterectomy has a great symbolic importance to many women. The first kind of study is often done by gynecologists soon after the operation, and the second kind of approach is taken by psychoanalytically trained (such as "Freudian") psychiatrists. It seems to me that both are correct. Hysterectomy does have an important symbolic significance to most of us at some level, and most of us adjust to it well.

What can you, as a person who may have a hysterectomy or who is close to someone who may have a hysterectomy, learn from all of these research studies?

1. The research is not conclusive. It does not prove that hysterectomy is always trouble-free or that hysterectomy is always

devastating. Anyone who tells you the research proves one way or the other is speaking from his or her own biases.

2. Most women do not have *major* psychological problems after hysterectomy.

3. Women are more likely to have psychological problems after hysterectomy than after other kinds of surgery, and are more likely to have problems after hysterectomy than if they have no operation.

One good follow-up study done by a gynecologist is that of Bruce C. Richards, M.D., of Lakewood, Colorado, entitled "Hysterectomy: From Women to Women," published in the *American Journal of Obstetrics and Gynecology* on June 15, 1978. Richards sent a questionnaire to 340 women who had had hysterectomies in 1975. He wanted to show that his patients, who were generally well informed, perceived their hysterectomies to be elective in the sense that they were not done for major illness or life-threatening conditions, and yet the women are glad they had hysterectomies.

Richards was concerned about patronizing gynecologists or "avant-garde libbers" who tell women what they should do. Richards' informed-consent form appears to be very thorough, and the first sentence states that the mortality rate of hysterectomy is 16.4 per 10,000. The consent form discusses other complications and emphasizes the elective nature of the hysterectomy.

The questionnaire sent to the women who had had hysterectomies in 1975 found very positive results. Over 90 percent of the women said that they were pleased they had had a hysterectomy. Most would encourage a friend to proceed with rather than postpone a hysterectomy. When fully recovered, over 90 percent felt better or partly better and partly worse than before, and the ways they felt better included less inconvenience (69 percent), more energy (54 percent), better sex life (38 percent), and no more (or less) pain (15 percent). Only a small portion answered about ways they felt worse, and those included weight gain (9 percent), worse sex life (6 percent), and depression and weight loss. Richards asked whether women perceived their hysterectomy to have been elective. Almost 70 percent said yes. He then asked whether, if their hysterectomy had been elective, they thought it was unnecessary. Over 90 percent said no, it had not been unnecessary. In addition, over 90 percent of the women said they were aware of the risks inherent in hysterectomy. He asked whether they had felt they needed a second opinion to help them decide to have the surgery, and whether they had had one. About a third said they needed a second opinion, slightly more said they sought a second opinion, and over half said no to both questions.

Richards has done an appropriate and responsible study. His major point was that the woman, not the physician, should be given information in order to make an informed decision. He objects to statements such as Ralph C. Wright's that the uterus is a useless organ. I would judge that his procedures for informing women of the risks of hysterectomy are good.

Nevertheless, there is a lot we do not learn from a study such as this. We do not know how the dynamics of the doctor–patient relationship work. How can we separate the attitudes of the doctor from the response of his or her patient? These are patients from Richards' medical group, and his own assumptions about surgery will have a major impact on them. In a footnote he mentions that there were three cases "in which the gynecologist felt that because of significant personality clash it would be unwise to send the questionnaire." That is, of course, a very small number, and yet those are angry women whose voices are not heard in his study. Also, the title of his article is misleading. It is called "Hysterectomy: From Women to Women," yet it is written by a male doctor and published in a medical journal.

Another very well-known study shows very different results. D. H. Richards, a British general practitioner, has done a series of studies that identify what he called a posthysterectomy syndrome. In the first study two hundred women who had had a hysterectomy were identified, and then two hundred female patients' records were selected as being similar to those of the hysterectomy patients', but with no hysterectomy (controls). The records of all the women were then searched to see whether any had sought help for depression from their doctors. Richards defined depression for the purpose of his study as a condition treated by specific antidepressive drugs.

The study showed that women who have had hysterectomies are four times more likely to become depressed within three years of the operation than women who have not had hysterectomies. Richards found that the depression in women who have had hysterectomies was longer and more severe than in a control group, and that some of them were admitted to mental hospitals within three years of the operation. He also found that whether the woman had had children and whether her ovaries had been removed had little effect on the chances she would become depressed, but that her age did have an influence. Depression was higher among younger women.

This was also the first study to point out that many women have hot flashes after hysterectomy, even when their ovaries have not been removed. Richards speculated that an endocrine factor might be involved in hysterectomy itself.

He identified three groups of women who are "at risk for depression after hysterectomy": women who are under forty; women who had no abnormality at the operation, that is, women who had the operation for conditions other than cancer; and women who had had depression before the hysterectomy. This last statement has been interpreted by many to mean that women seek out hysterectomy because of their neurotic difficulties. This, of course, may be true, but I believe a fairer interpretation is that women who have dealt with stress by becoming depressed at other times in their life are more likely to become depressed after hysterectomy than women who have dealt with stress in other ways.

Based on criticisms of this study, Richards did a second study. In this one he compared women who had had hysterectomy with women who had had other surgery, in order to separate the effects of surgery itself from the effects of hysterectomy. Richards further suspected that the hysterectomy patients were probably more closely followed by their doctors because they had had surgery, so mild depression might have been more visible than in women who had had no operation and might have had fewer doctor visits.

In this second study Richards designed a questionnaire, and each woman was visited and interviewed. If a woman said she had been depressed, her medical records were searched to see whether she had sought help or been treated for depression by her doctor. The study showed that both depression that the woman felt but did not seek help for and depression as treated by doctors were far more common among women who had had hysterectomies than among women who had had other operations. Approximately 70 percent of the hysterectomy patients were depressed within three years of their operations, while only 30 percent of the other women had been depressed. Also, when a woman was treated for depression after hysterectomy, the treatment went on for a longer time, approximately a year on the average. In the control group a woman was treated for approximately four months. Again in this study, more women had been treated for depression before hysterectomy than before other surgeries, but when all women who had been treated for depression before their surgery were eliminated from the study, there was still significantly more posthysterectomy depression than depression after other operations. Richards identified headaches, a particular kind of fatigue, and dizziness as more common after hysterectomy. In addition, the women reported the length of time it took before they felt fully normal. The average reported by hysterectomy patients was nearly one year, while those having other operations said that they were back to normal in about three months.

In terms of sexual feelings the American Richards' study reported overwhelmingly better sexual response. The British Richards found no consistent effects. Of the patients in his study who had not had hysterectomies, by far the major portion had unchanged libido or sexual appetite. Of the hysterectomy group, eleven reported improved libido, twenty-one reduced libido, and fifteen were unchanged. An interesting comment on the assumptions about women's sexual activity is that one category under sexual experience was "not applicable (widows, spinsters)." I know many widows and spinsters who do remain sexually active in one way or another!

The contrast between these two studies probably reflects some cultural variation in the way that women cope with stress, and in their willingness to "admit" depression. It also represents contrasts between two medical systems. In the American system the woman has sought out the gynecologist and paid him (or her insurance company has paid him). The British general practitioners are following up on women for whom they may have recommended a consultation by a gynecologist, but the doctors derive no financial gain from doing the surgery.

Attitudes and feelings are so intertwined with social situations that it is not surprising that patients of an American gynecologist would answer differently from patients in the British study. Also, the American study questioned women within a year or so after their surgery. Many of D. H. Richards' findings of depression were in the second year after hysterectomy and sometimes even later than that.

We can also learn a great deal from the classic studies of psychoanalytic implications of hysterectomy.

One of the most famous is a study entitled "The Psychologic Importance of the Uterus and Its Functions," published in 1958 by Marvin G. Drellich and Irving Bieber. This study involved a random selection of twenty-three patients who were to have hysterectomies. They were interviewed at length before the operation and during their hospital stay, and were followed for six to twelve months after surgery.

Some comments in the article sound strange or offensive to our ears today. But the article contains a wealth of information from women concerning their feelings about their uteruses and about hysterectomy. The authors organized their findings into several functions of the uterus. They found that for many of the women they interviewed, the uterus had an important reproductive function. Women who had not completed the childbearing that they wanted felt a great sense of loss. The authors say:

It is clear, then, that the ability to have children and the bearing and raising of children serves a variety of needs and functions in the adaptation of different women. For some it is consciously valued as a source of pleasure and fulfillment, for others it is verbalized as a necessary concession to men, an act of giving which satisfies the husband's paternal needs, or his "conceit" or both. For some women, even though they desired no more children, the knowledge that they were able to bear children gave them the feeling of being complete and feminine and the loss of childbearing ability was viewed as rendering a woman something less than a complete female.

Drellich and Bieber also found that menstruation was important to the women they interviewed, even when their periods had been painful. They valued menstruation for cleansing, or for part of the "rhythm of life." Some women before the surgery were concerned about their general health after the hysterectomy. They saw the uterus as a source of strength, health, and general effectiveness. Many of them spoke of experiences similar to those documented by D. H. Richards, though explaining their slow recovery with phrases such as "It may sound silly but I believe your strength comes from your womanly organ."

The sexual function of the uterus was very important for fifteen of the women Drellich and Bieber interviewed. The changes that the women experienced were not consistent, but many of them both anticipated changes in sexual feelings and experienced changes afterward. It is interesting that in this study in 1958, women expressed to the researchers sexual experiences and feelings that Masters and Johnson later documented (in 1966) as physiologically based. However, Drellich and Bieber interpreted the experiences as psychological in nature. For example, here is a description of a woman in their study:

One forty year old patient clearly illustrated her concept of the uterus as her "sex organ." Her husband had been partly disabled by a chronic neurologic disease and had made very infrequent sexual overtures to her for several years. Her chief complaint to the gynecologist was a feeling of swelling, distension and pressure in her mid-abdominal region. She consciously visualized her uterus as having the characteristics of an "internal penis." She felt that the intermittent distension of her abdomen was caused by her uterus becoming swollen and erect due to sexual desire. Because of her husband's indifference to her sexual needs and her reluctance to seek an alternative sexual outlet, she felt that her uterus remained engorged and turgid, allegedly returning to normal only after her infrequent sexual intercourse with her husband. She stated, "If I were a man, I'd be walking around with a big penis all the time."

That woman is describing accurately the experience of sexual excitement causing the uterus to become engorged with blood, and causing pelvic discomfort until relieved by orgasm. Masters and Johnson have described women who experienced considerable pain from this.

Another area Drellich and Bieber's subjects described is the reaction of men to women's surgery. They sometimes find that men are less interested, or are concerned that they will injure the woman.

For some women the disease for which they had the hysterectomy was seen as a punishment for activities about which they felt guilty. As in the discussion of sexuality, the women frequently expressed ideas that are now accepted as part of "holistic health," while at the time of the article they were seen as exclusively psychological.

Drellich and Bieber end their article with a plea for acknowledging the importance of the uterus in women's psychological experiences as being similar to the importance of the penis for men. Although totally lacking today's feminist language, this article is recommended for its respectful presentation of women's experience.

A very different approach to research about psychiatric illness after hysterectomy was taken by Montague Barker in an article in the *British Medical Journal* of April 13, 1968. Barker worked in the Department of Psychiatry at the University of Dundee, Scotland. Because there is a national health service in Scotland, he had access to centralized records of all women who had had operations in that area. His study was a statistical one, comparing the rates of psychiatric referral of women who had had hysterectomy with women who had had cholecystectomy, or gallbladder removal, and the predicted rate of psychiatric referral in the general population. Psychiatric referral in the United Kingdom means that the person's general practitioner has referred the person to a psychiatrist for additional treatment. That kind of referral is done more frequently in the British system, since the referring general practitioner loses no money by referring a patient on to a specialist.

The study included the records of all 729 women who had undergone a hysterectomy in the city of Dundee in the years 1960 through 1964. The comparison group, all women who had had a cholecystectomy, included 280 people. The psychiatric records were then searched up to the end of 1966, which means that the patients were followed for between two and seven years after their operations.

The study showed that a significantly higher proportion of women who had had a hysterectomy than women who had had a cholecystectomy were referred to a psychiatrist after their operation. The numbers are still quite small. Only 7 percent of the women after hysterectomy were referred to a psychiatrist. Of those who had never been referred to a psychiatrist before the operation, only 5 percent were referred to a psychiatrist after hysterectomy. Nevertheless, the proportion of women who were referred after cholecystectomy was far smaller. Comparing women who were referred to psychiatrists after hysterectomy with those who might have been referred from the general population, the figures showed that about the same number were referred after a cholecystectomy as you might expect in the general population, but a far higher proportion was referred after hysterectomy. There was no significant difference statistically between women whose ovaries had been removed and women whose ovaries had not been removed in terms of psychiatric referral.

Barker's figures also showed that those women who had had hysterectomy for severe indications, such as cancer or severe fibroids or anemia, had a lower referral rate than those who had no physical abnormality. This is partly because those women who had a hysterectomy with no physical abnormality had been more likely to have had psychiatric referral before their hysterectomies. A finding such as this is frequently explained by saying it is neurotic women who seek out unnecessary hysterectomy, and that is the reason they have a higher rate of depression after surgery. But in a medical system where no satisfactory relief of a woman's emotional problems is available, and where the system pushes toward hysterectomy, it seems wrong to blame the woman for choosing hysterectomy as a last desperate attempt.

Another factor related to referral to a psychiatrist was marital disruption. Barker's figures suggest that hysterectomy patients were no more likely to be divorced than other women, but of those referred to a psychiatrist after the operation, far more had undergone marital disruption than had been in a stable marriage. To health professionals this should suggest that if they know a woman is undergoing marital stress, they should be especially alert to her emotional needs.

Barker's figures show that the incidence of psychiatric referral among the 10 percent of women who had never been married was the same as for married women. In addition, there was no significant difference between women who had had children and women who had not. Barker's figures showed that for the married women who were referred to psychiatrists, a significant proportion of the men showed "disturbed behavior after the hysterectomy, including impotence, suicide, irritability, promiscuity, and taunting the wife with being 'only half a woman' or 'no use.'"

The largest number of women who were referred to psychiatrists had a diagnosis of depression. Twenty-eight percent of the patients had been admitted to a general hospital having taken an overdose of drugs "while depressed in spirits."

Barker also shows that often emotional problems do not show up in the immediate postoperative period. Many of the women in his study stated that they felt better during the period immediately after the surgery, and their symptoms of depression occurred in the end of the first year or during the second year after their operation. Barker concludes his article with some suggestions to gynecologists, that they be very cautious about performing a hysterectomy on a woman who has a previous history of emotional difficulty, and that they follow up with a general practitioner for a period of two years after a hysterectomy, being alert to signs of depression.

We have seen examples of three kinds of studies, questionnaires given out by the gynecologist, in-depth studies by psychoanalysts, and statistical studies. Another group of studies are reviews of literature, often done by psychologists. The most significant of these, and the only major studies of hysterectomy done by women, are by Niles Newton of Northwestern University and her associates. They come to the following conclusions:

> Elective hysterectomy has become culturally patterned as a normal part of the life cycle with more than half of all American women destined for hysterectomy if current rates continue. In keeping with this widespread acceptance, both women and their doctors frequently express satisfaction with the operation. Those sequelae that do occur appear to be serious in only a few women, though more minor disturbances do appear in a sizable number. Repeated or controlled studies indicate that hysterectomy may yield problems for some women in the following areas: rejection by male partners, hot flushes after conservation of ovarian tissue, severe hot flushes after ovariectomy, long time psychourinary problems, weight changes, lingering fatigue and prolonged convalescence, painful intercourse, depression,

sleep disturbances, and other psychiatric symptoms. Prospective studies using mixed control groups are needed which follow patients at least two years post-operatively, as repeated studies have shown "sleeper effect" after hysterectomy with sequelae developing after the first six months or even after one year.

SOURCE NOTES

CHAPTER 2

Page
No.
12. The percentages for the various causes of hysterectomy discussed in this chapter are based on a review by Koepsell of large studies by Ledger and Child and others. The references are:

> Thomas Koepsell et al. "Prevalance of Prior Hysterectomy in the Seattle-Tacoma Area." *American Journal of Public Health* 70:1 (Jan. 1980):40–47.
> W.J. Ledger and M.A. Child. "The Hospital Care of Patients Undergoing Hysterectomy: An Analysis of 12,026 Patients from the Professional Activity Study." *American Journal of Obstetrics and Gynecology* 117 (1973):423–433.

13. *Fibroids.* Good information on fibroids is included in the following:

> Lucienne Lanson. *From Woman to Woman.* New York: Knopf, 1978.
> R.W. Kistner. *Gynecology: Principles and Practice.* 2nd ed. Chicago: Yearbook Medical Publishers, 1971.

13. *black women get fibroids.* Kistner reports the incidence is three to nine times higher in black women. Kistner, p. 226.

14. *subserous fibroid.* Kistner, p. 226, and figures attached.

14. *with a uterine weight of over 200 grams.* Frank J. Dyck et al. "Effect of Surveillance on the Number of Hysterectomies in the Province of Saskatchewan." *New England Journal of Medicine* 296:23 (June 9, 1977):1326–28.

14. *sixteen weeks of pregnancy.* Kistner, p. 232.

14. *"uh, most likely . . ."* Diana Scully. *Men Who Control Women's Health.* Boston: Houghton Mifflin, 1980, p. 232.

15. *myomectomy.* Kistner, p. 232.

16. *specialist on infertility.* A book that is a very good resource is Mary Harrison. *Infertility: A Couple's Guide to It's Causes.* Boston: Houghton Mifflin, 1979.

16. *a recently introduced surgical treatment.* "Hysterectomies Avoided with New Surgical Techniques." *Modern Medicine* (Aug. 15– Sept. 15, 1980).

17. *Endometriosis.* Good references on endometriosis are:

> *Important Facts About Endometriosis.* Patient Information Booklet. American College of Obstetrics and Gynecologists, 1979.
> *Endometriosis and Its Treatment.* Handout from Resolve, Inc. Available from PO Box 474, Belmont, MA 02718.
> Clara Valverde. "*Endometriosis: Healing with the Mind's Eye.*" *Healthsharing: A Canadian Women's Health Quarterly* (Spring 1981):13.

19. *danazol.* Advantages of danazol are described by Dr. Robert Greenblatt. Risks are described in leaflet by Resolve.

> R.B. Greenblatt and V. Tzingounis. "Danazol Treatment of Endometriosis: Long Term Follow-up." *Fertility and Sterilization* 32 (Nov. 1979):518–520.
> *Endometriosis and Its Treatment.* Leaflet from Resolve, Inc.

22. *the risk of PID is estimated.* Ronald T. Burkman. "Intrauterine Device Use and the Risk of Pelvic Inflammatory Disease." *American Journal of Obstetrics and Gynecology* 138:7, Part 2 (Dec. 1, 1980).

23. *Acute PID.* A good summary of recent information on PID is available from the Women and Health Roundtable, 2000 P Street, NW, Suite 403, Washington, D.C., 20036. *The Roundtable Report*, Vol. IV, No. 9 (Oct. 1980) reviews work by James W. Curran.

24. *By the year 2000.* Curran in *Roundtable Report*. Additional papers are available from James W. Curran, M.D., Venereal Disease Control Division, Center for Disease Control, Atlanta, GA 30333.

26. *perhaps 14 to 29 percent.* Thomas Koepsell et al. "Prevalence of Prior Hysterectomy in the Seattle-Tacoma Area." *American Journal of Public Health* 70:1 (Jan. 1980):40–47.

30. *Diagnosis is difficult.* Kistner, p. 225.

30. *Although 8 to 20 percent of hysterectomy patients.* Kistner, p. 221.

31. *vitamin A deficiency.* "Vitamin A for Heavy Menstrual Bleeding." *Prevention* (June 1977).

32. *Norma Swenson.* Personal communication (March 30, 1981).

33. *8 to 12 percent.* Thomas Koepsell et al. "Prevalence of Prior Hysterectomy in the Seattle-Tacoma Area." *American Journal of Public Health* 70:1 (Jan. 1980):40–47.

34. Table source: Robert C. Knapp et al. "Gynecologic Cancer." *Cancer: A Manual for Practitioners.* 5th ed. Boston: American Cancer Society, Massachusetts Division, 1978.

34. *there is a higher rate.* Knapp.

35. Table source: James G. Blythe. "What to Do about the Patient with an Abnormal Pap Smear." *Modern Medicine* (Feb. 15, 1978).

36. *One study.* M. Brudnell et al. "The Management of Dysplasia, Carcinoma in Situ and Microcarcinoma of the Cervix." *Journal of Obstetrics and Gynecology of the British Commonwealth* 80:8 (1973):673–679. (Cited by Gena Corea)

37. *caused by a virus.* Knapp.

38. *1 percent of cancer cases.* Boston Women's Health Book Collective, *Our Bodies, Ourselves,* New York: Simon and Schuster, 1976.

39. *Carl and Stephanie Simonton.* Carl Simonton et al. *Getting Well Again.* New York: Bantam, 1980.

ADDITIONAL REFERENCES FOR CHAPTER 2 PROBLEMS & ALTERNATIVES

"The Nulliparous Patient, the IUD, and Subsequent Fertility." *British Medical Journal* (July 22, 1978).

"Women's Trials in IUD Suit: 'Were you a cocktail or a food waitress?' " *CARASA News* 2:10 (Nov. 1978).

Caress, Barbara. "Sterilization: Women Fit to Be Tied." *Health/Pac Bulletin.* No. 62 (Jan.–Feb. 1975).

Clark, Charles C.,et al. "CO_2 Embolus: Serious Complication of Laparoscopy." *Modern Medicine* (Jan. 30, 1978).

Cooper, Kenneth H. *The New Aerobics.* New York: Bantam, 1970.

Dietz, Jean. "Two Studies Support Cancer Self-Exams." *Boston Globe* (Aug. 10, 1978).

Dippel, Louis A. "The Role of Hysterectomy in the Production of Menopausal Symptoms." *American Journal of Obstetrics and Gynecology* 37:1 (Jan. 1939):110–113.

Donsback, Kurt W. *Menopause.* Pamphlet by International Institute of Natural Health Sciences, P.O. Box 5550, Huntington Beach, CA 92646.

Gifford-Jones, W. *What Every Woman Should Know about Hysterectomy.* New York: Funk and Wagnalls, 1977.

Medical Self-Care, Box 718, Inverness, CA 94937.

"Three Studies Link Pelvic Abscesses to IUD's." *OB-GYN Observer* (June 1977).

Porter, Cedric W., and Jaroslav F. Hulka. "Female Sterilization in Current Clinical Practice." *Family Planning Perspective* 6:1 (Winter 1974):30–38.

Project of the Federation of Organizations for Professional Women. "The Role of the Food and Drug Administration in Assuring That IUD Patient Labeling Information Will Be Distributed." Report No. 8. Women and Health Roundtable, 2000 P Street, NW, Washington, D.C. 20036.

CHAPTER 3

Page
No.
42. *unpublished data.* National Center for Health Statistics, Hospital Discharge Survey (April 9, 1981).

42. *50 percent.* John P. Bunker. "Elective Hysterectomy: Pro and Con." *New England Journal of Medicine* 295:5 (July 29, 1976).

42. *62 percent.* Bruce C. Richards. "Hysterectomy: From Women to Women." *American Journal of Obstetrics and Gynecology* 131:4 (June 15, 1978):446–452.

43. *Center for Disease Control.* Center for Disease Control. *Surgical Sterilization Surveillance Hysterectomy in Women Aged 15–44,* U.S. Department of Health and Human Services: Public Health Service, Sept. 1980.

43. *National Center for Health Statistics* (1979). Unpublished data, National Center for Health Statistics, Hospital Discharge Survey (April 9, 1981).

43. *personal communication.* National Center for Health Statistics (Oct. 1978).

43. *1976 and 1975.* Abraham Ranofsky. "Utilization of Short-Stay Hospitals: Annual Summary for the United States, 1976." *Vital*

and Health Statistics. Series 13, No. 37, DHEW Publication No. (PHS) 78-1788.

43. *decline of 17 percent*. Thomas Koepsell et al. "Prevalence of Prior Hysterectomy in the Seattle-Tacoma Area." *American Journal of Public Health* 70:1 (Jan. 1980):45.

43. *One large study in 1980.* Koepsell.

43. *health insurance*. Joann Rodgers. "Rush to Surgery." *New York Times Magazine* (Sept. 21, 1975):34; Letters (Oct. 12, 1975).

43. *higher income*. Koepsell.

43. *fee-for-service basis*. Rodgers.

44. *vary with the part of the country*. J. Wennberg and A. Gittelsohn. "Small area variations in Health Care Delivery." *Science* 182 (1973):1102–1108.

44. *rose 742 percent*. Lester T. Hibbard. "Sexual sterilization by elective hysterectomy." *American Journal of Obstetrics and Gynecology* 112:8 (April 1972):1076–1083.

44. *vary with the time of the year*. Norma Swenson, Boston's Women's Health Book Collective. Personal communication.

44. *health plan required*. E.G. McCarthy and G.W. Widmer. "Effects of Screening by Consultants on Recommended Elective Surgical Procedures, *New England Journal of Medicine*, 291:1331 (1974).

44. *Saskatchewan*. Frank J. Dyck et al. "Effects of Surveillance on the Number of Hysterectomies in the Province of Saskatchewan." *New England Journal of Medicine* 296:23 (June 9, 1977).

44. *stimulate fibroids*. Barbara Seaman and Gideon Seaman. *Women and the Crisis in Sex Hormones*. New York: Rawson, 1977; New York: Bantam, 1978 (paper).

45. *"Some of us aren't making a living. . ."* Joann Rodgers. "Rush to Surgery." *New York Times Magazine* (Sept. 21, 1975):34; letters section (Oct. 12, 1975).

46. *"The uterus has but one function . . ."* Ralph C. Wright. "Hysterectomy: Past, Present, and Future." *Obstetrics and Gynecology* 33:4 (April 1968):560–563.

48. *In Britain.* "What Every Woman Needs to Know." Editorial in *Lancet* (Jan. 29, 1977):8005.

48. *the Subcommittee . . . held major hearings.* House of Representatives Subcommittee on Oversights and Investigations. "Cost and Quality of Health Care: Unnecessary Surgery." Ninety-fourth Congress, Second Session (Jan. 1976):30–34.

50. *"We were deliberately liberal . . ."* Testimony by Dr. Frank Dyck, Hearing on Unnecessary Surgery. Hysterectomy Case Study. Assembly, California Legislature, Committee on Health, Los Angeles, California (Dec. 12, 1979).

50. *list of indications.* Frank J. Dyck et al. "Effect of Surveillance on the Number of Hysterectomies in the Province of Saskatchewan." *The New England Journal of Medicine* 296:23 (June 9, 1977): 1326–28.

50. *Some doctors.* Boston Women's Health Book Collective. *Our Bodies, Ourselves.* New York: Simon and Schuster, 1979.

51. *In one study of the second-opinion program.*

   Eugene G. McCarthy, testimony before House Hearings on May 2, 1977, Vol. 1, page 157.
   Hearings before the Subcommittee on Oversight and Investigation of the Committee on Interstate and Foreign Commerce, U.S. House of Representatives. *Cost and Quality of Surgical Care.* Vol. 1 (Serial No. 95–32). 1978; Vol. 2 (Serial No. 95–63), 1978.

53. *Tubal ligation itself.* Karen Wynn. "Second Thoughts about Sterilization." *Sister* (newspaper), 1977; reprints are 25¢ from 250 Howard Ave., New Haven, Conn. 06519.

53. *Compared to tubal ligation.* Deborah Larned. "The Greening of the Womb." *New Times Magazine* (Dec. 12, 1974):35–39.

54. *Philip Cole.* Philip Cole and Joyce Berlin. "Elective Hysterectomy." *American Journal of Obstetrics and Gynecology* 129:2 (Sept. 1977):117–123.

54. *James H. Sammons.* James H. Sammons. Testimony, House Hearings on Costs and Quality of Surgery, Vol. I (May 9, 1977).

54. *Ralph C. Wright.* Ralph Wright. "Elective Hysterectomy: Letters to the Editor." *Obstetrics and Gynecology* 34:4 (Oct. 1969): 626–627.

55. *At its 1971 anuual meeting.* Barbara Caress. "Womb-Bomb." *Health/Pac Bulletin* (July–Aug. 1977):13–14.

56. *60,000 men.* Leonard Zinman et al. *Carcinoma of the Prostate and Bladder in Cancer: A Manual for Practitioners.* 5th ed. Boston: American Cancer Society Massachusetts Division. 1978.

56. *cervical cancer.* Robert C. Knapp et al. "Gynecologic Cancer." *Cancer: A Manual for Practitioners.* 5th ed. Boston: American Cancer Society Massachusetts Division, 1978.

57. *The death rate.* John P. Bunker et al. "Elective Hysterectomy: Pro and Con." *New England Journal of Medicine* 295:5 (July 29, 1976):264–268.

57. *Hormone levels may be affected.*

> Sergio Stone et al. "The Acute Effect of Hysterectomy on Ovarian Function." *American Journal of Obstetrics and Gynecology* 121:2 (Jan. 15, 1975):193–197.
> Brooks Ranney and Samir Abu-Ghazaleh. "The Future Function and Fortune of Ovarian Tissue Which is Retained in vivo during Hysterectomy." *American Journal of Obstetrics and Gynecology.* Vol. 128, No. 6 (July 15, 1977):626–634.

HELPFUL REFERENCES FOR CHAPTER 3

The following references have also been helpful in preparing this chapter:

Adamson, Lesley. "Hysterectomy." *The Guardian* (England) (June 13, 1978).
Brody, Jane E. "Blue Cross Acts to Limit Surgery." *New York Times* (March 16, 1976):1.

Bunker, John P. et al. *Costs, Risks and Benefits of Surgery*. New York: Oxford University Press, 1977.

Bunker, John P. "Surgical Manpower: A Comparison of Operations and Surgeons in the United States and in England and Wales." *New England Journal of Medicine* 282:3 (Jan. 15, 1970):135–143.

Bunker, John P. Testimony, Hearings on Quality of Surgical Care. Vol. I. U.S. House of Representatives Subcommittee on Oversight and Investigations, Serial No. 95–32 (1977).

Burchell, R. Clay. "Decision Regarding Hysterectomy." *American Journal of Obstetrics and Gynecology* 127:2 (Jan. 1977):113–117.

Caress, Barbara. "Sterilization: Women Fit to Be Tied." *Health/Pac. Bulletin* 62 (Jan.–Feb. 1975):1–13.

Cohen, Marcia. "Needless Hysterectomies." *Ladies Home Journal* (March 1976):88–92.

Cohn, Victor. "U.S. Moves to Curb Unneeded Surgery." *Washington Post* (Nov. 2, 1977).

Deane, Robert T. and Arthur Ulene. "Hysterectomy or Tubal Ligation for Sterilization: A Cost-Effectiveness Analysis." *Inquiry*. Vol. XIV, (March 1977):73.

Emerson, Ralph S. and John J. Creedon. "Unjustified Surgery Dilemma." *New York State Journal of Medicine* 77:5 (April 1977):779–785.

Hibbard, Lester T. "Sexual Sterilization by Elective Hysterectomy." *American Journal of Obstetrics and Gynecology* 112:8 (April 15, 1972):1076–1083.

Jackson, M., et al. "Elective Hysterectomy: A Cost-Benefit Analysis." *Inquiry* 15 (1978):275–280.

Kotulak, Ronald. "Hysterectomies Needed, Wanted—M.D." *Chicago Tribune* (July 5, 1978).

Landesman, Robert. "Elective Hysterectomy" (Letter to the Editor). *Obstetrics and Gynecology* 34:4 (Oct. 1969):625–626.

Langer, Alvin, et al. "Comparison of Sterilization by Tubal Ligation and Hysterectomy." *Surgery, Gynecology and Obstetrics*. 140:2 (Feb. 1975):235–238.

Ledger, William J., and Margaret A. Child. "The Hospital Care of Patients Undergoing Hysterectomy: An Analysis of 12,026 Patients from the Professional Activity Study." *American Journal of Obstetrics and Gynecology* 117:3 (Oct. 1973):423–433.

Lembke, Paul A. "Medical Auditing by Scientific Methods." *JAMA* 167:7 (Oct. 13, 1956):646–655.

Levinson, Carl J. "Hysterectomy Complications." *Clinical Obstetrics and Gynecology* (Sept. 15, 1972):802–826.

Lewis, Charles E. "Variations in the Incidence of Surgery." *The New England Journal of Medicine* 281:16 (Oct. 1969):880–884.

Little, William A. "Current Aspects of Sterilization: The Selection and

Application of Various Surgical Methods of Sterilization." *American Journal of Obstetrics and Gynecology* 123:1 (Sept. 1, 1975):12–18.

LoGerfo, James P. "Variations in Surgical Rates: Fact Versus Fantasy." *The New England Journal of Medicine* 297:7 (Aug. 18, 1977):387–389.

LoGerfo, J. Petal. "Rates of Surgical Care in Prepaid Group Practices and the Independent Settings: What Are the Reasons for the Difference?" *Medical Care* 17:1–10 (1979).

McCann, Margaret F. and Elton Kessel. "Late Effects of Female Sterilization." *The Lancet* (Jan. 7, 1978).

———. National Center for Health Statistics. Monthly Vital Statistics Reports. *Surgery in Short Stay Hospitals: U.S., 1973.* 24:3 (May 30, 1975).

"Operation Defended as Patient's Choice." *Washington Post* (July 6, 1978).

———. U.S. Dept. of HEW, Surgical Operations in Short Stay Hospitals, (United States 1971), Vital and Health Statistics, 12:18, Nov. 1974, (DHEW), Pub. #75–1769.

Parrott, Max H. "Elective Hysterectomy." *American Journal of Obstetrics and Gynecology* 113:4 (June 1972):531–540.

Paulshock, B.Z. " 'Unnecessary' Surgery: Who'll Have the Final Say?" *Medical Economics* (March 7, 1977):75–80.

Pratt, Joseph H. "Common Complications of Vaginal Hysterectomy: Thoughts Regarding Their Prevention and Management." *Clinical Obstetrics and Gynecology* 19:3 (Sept. 1976):645–659.

Rosenfeld, Bernard, et al. *A Health Research Group Study on Surgical Sterilization: Present Abuses and Proposed Regulations.* Washington, D.C.: Health Research Group, (Oct. 29, 1973).

Sammons, James H. Testimony, House Hearings on Costs and Quality of Surgery. Vol. 1 (May 9, 1977).

Schulman, Harold. "Major Surgery for Abortion and Sterilization." *Obstetrics and Gynecology* 40:5 (Nov. 1972):738–739.

Sloan, Don. "Elective Hysterectomy" (Letter to the Editor). *Obstetrics and Gynecology* 34:4 (Oct. 1969):626.

Synmonds, Richard E. "Ureteral Injuries Associated with Gynecologic Surgery: Prevention and Management." *Clinical Obstetrics and Gynecology* 19:3 (Sept. 1976):623–645.

Walker, A.M., and H. Jick. "Temporal and Regional Variations in Hysterectomy Rates in the United States, 1970–1975." *American Journal of Epidemiology* 110 (1979):41–46.

Wolfe, Sidney M. and Robert E. McGarrah, Jr. Letter to Caspar W. Weinberger, *Health Research Group* (Feb. 5, 1974).

Wright, R.C. "Hysterectomy: Past, Present and Future." *Obstetrics and Gynecology* 33 (1969):560–563.

ADDITIONAL REFERENCES FOR CHAPTER 3
RATES & RISKS

Barker-Benfield, G.J. "A Historical Perspective on Women's Health Care–Female Circumcision." *Women and Health* 1:1 (Jan. 1976): 13–20.

Burden, Friedlander, et al. (Introduced by). *A Local Law . . . No. 37.* Local Law of the City of New York for the Year 1977, No. 37.

Farrell, William E. "AMA Scores 'Unneeded Surgery' Report." *New York Times* (May 12, 1976).

Fifer, William R. et al. "Whither Went the Issues? (An Audit of Hysterectomy for Leiomyoma)." *Quality Review Bulletin* (March 1977):12.

Friedman, Stanley, "Elective Hysterectomy." Letter to the Editor, *Obstetrics and Gynecology* 34:4 (Oct. 1969):625.

"HEW Urges Patients to Get Second Opinion Before Elective Surgery." *Los Angeles Times* (Nov. 2, 1977):15.

Higgin, J.R. "More Hysterectomies—Fact, Fantasy, or Fad?" *The Canadian Nurse* 67:7 (July 1971):33–37.

Hume, Ellen. "Hysterectomies to 'Relieve Anxiety' Advocated." *Los Angeles Times* 24, Pt. I (May 10, 1977).

"Hysterectomy of the Poor: Feds on Trail of Abuses." *Medical Tribune* (July 5, 1978).

Jenkins,Van R., II. "Unnecessary—Elective—Indicated? Audit Criteria of the American College of Obstetricians and Gynecologists to Assess Abdominal Hysterectomy for Uterine Leiomyoma." *Quality Review Bulletin* (May 1977):7.

Lyon, Joseph L. and John W. Gardner. "The Rising Frequency of Hysterectomy: Its Effect on Uterine Cancer Rates." *American Journal of Epidemiology.* Vol. 105, No. 5 (1977):439–443.

Mintz, Morton. "Patients to get FDA-ordered brochure on hazards of IUD." *Washington Post* (Nov. 5, 1977).

Roos, Noralou P., et al. "Elective Surgery Rates—Do High Rates Mean Lower Standards?" *The New England Journal of Medicine* 297:7 (Aug. 18, 1977):360–65.

Rosenfeld, Bernard, et al. *A Health Research Group Study on Surgical Sterilization: Present Abuses and Proposed Regulations.* Washington, D.C.: Health Research Group (Oct. 29, 1973).

Rosenbaum, David E. "HEW to Issue New Regulations to Prevent Forced Sterilizations." *New York Times* (Dec. 2, 1977).

Scully, Diana H. "Women and Unnecessary Gynecological Surgery." Unpublished paper read at the American Sociological Association Convention, September 1976.

Shanahan, Maryanne "Without Fruition: Critique of a Nursing Audit of Hysterectomy." *Quality Review Bulletin* (March 1977):18.

"Sterilization Controls Upheld in California Court." ACOG *Newsletter* (June 1978).

"Sterilization Abuse to Be Studied." *Association for Voluntary Sterilization News* (June 1978).

"Sterilization Rate Rising." *Boston Globe* (April 17, 1978).

"Sterilization Use Still on the Rise." *Association for Voluntary Sterilization News* (June 1978).

"Surgical Sterilization Gaining Popularity." *Modern Medicine* (June 15–30, 1978).

Stern, Elizabeth, et al. "Pap Testing and Hysterectomy Prevalence: A Survey of Communities with High and Low Cervical Cancer Rates." *American Journal of Epidemiology.* Vol. 106, No. 4 (1977):296–305.

Stern, Elizabeth, "Papanicolaou Testing and Hysterectomy Prevalence in Low Income Communities: A Survey in Los Angeles County." Epidemiology and Cancer Registries in the Pacific Basin, Monograph 47, National Cancer Institute Monograph (1977).

Yogt, Thomas M. "Costs and Benefits of Hysterectomy." Correspondence Section, *The New England Journal of Medicine* 295:19, (Nov. 1976):1085.

CHAPTER 4

Page
No.

63. *con job.* This analogy is developed in Diana Scully. *Men Who Control Women's Health.* Boston: Houghton Mifflin, 1980.

63. *The sales pitch.* Scully, p. 224

65. *look back one hundred years.*

Barbara Ehrenreich and Deirdre English. *Complaints and Disorders: The Sexual Politics of Sickness.* Old Westbury, N.Y.: Feminist Press, 1973

Barbara Ehrenreich and Deirdre English. *For Her Own Good: One Hundred Years of the Experts' Advice to Women.* New York: Anchor, 1979.

Gena Corea's book *The Hidden Malpractice* also has exciting historical information; Gena Corea. *The Hidden Malpractice.* New York: Jove, 1977.

65. *Frederick Hollick.* Corea, p. 103.

65. *"She will prescribe . . ."* Corea, p. 103.

66. *Reproductive and mental organs.* Called "Psychology of the Ovary" by Ehrenreich and English (*Complaints and Disorders*).

66. *indigestion, insomnia.* Isaac Baker Brown, in an 1866 book cited by Corea, p. 108.

66. *Barker-Benfield.* Cited in Corea, p. 109.

68. *Irving Kenneth Zola.* Irving Kenneth Zola. "Medicine as an Institution of Social Control." *The Sociological Review* (new series). Vol. 20, No. 4 (Nov. 1972).

68. *Barbara Ehrenreich.* Barbara Ehrenreich and John Ehrenreich. "Health Care and Social Control." *Social Policy* (May–June 1974).

68. *Medicine is a system.* Barbara Ehrenreich. "Feminism and the Cultural Revolution in Health." Speech at the Conference on Women and Health, Boston, MA (April 4–7, 1975).

69. *"Mississippi appendectomy."* Deborah Larned. "The Greening of the Womb." *New Times Magazine* (Dec. 12, 1974):35–39.

70. *The increase in the number of hysterectomies.* Lester T. Hibbard. "Sexual Sterilization by Elective Hysterectomy." *American Journal of Obstetrics and Gynecology* 112:8 (April 1972):1076–1083.

70. *CARASA. Women Under Attack: Abortion, Sterilization Abuse and Reproductive Freedom.* New York: CARASA (Committee for Abortion Rights and Reproductive Freedom), 1979.

70. *CARASA cites a 1978 study*. CARASA, p. 51.

71. Table source. CARASA. Addendum, Figure 1, p. 4.

CHAPTER 5

**Page
No.**

79. *Gynecologists are trained*. Diana Scully. *Men Who Control Women's Health*. New York: Houghton Mifflin, 1980.

Other classic studies of medical school include:

> Howard S. Becker et al. *Boys in White*. University of Chicago Press, 1961.
> Howard S. Becker and Blanche Geer. "The Fate of Idealism in Medical School." *American Sociological Review* 28 (Feb. 1958):50–56.
> Eliot Friedson. *Profession of Medicine*. New York: Dodd, Mead, 1973.

79. *Doctors are trained*. Thanks to Marjorie Buck for this comment.

79. *Diana Scully*. Diana Scully. *Men Who Control Women's Health*, p. 221.

80. *patient's "social worth."* David Sudnow. "Dead on Arrival." *Transaction*. 5:1 (1967).

80. "*If like all human beings . . .*" Diana Scully and Pauline Bart. "A Funny Thing Happened on the Way to the Orifice: Women in Gynecology Textbooks." *American Journal of Sociology* 78:4 (1972):1048, citing C. Russell Scott. *The World of a Gynecologist* (1968):25.

80. *Norma Swenson*. (Personal communication)

ADDITIONAL REFERENCES FOR CHAPTER 5
WHAT'S A WOMAN TO DO?

Baciallei, Susan. "The Latest Medical News About—Hysterectomy." *Good Housekeeping* (Feb. 1976):17–77.

Ballard, L.A. "Gynecologic Surgery in the Aged." *Geriatrics* 24:4 (1969): 172–78.

Christ, J.E., and E.C. Lotze. "The Residual Ovary Syndrome." *Obstetrics and Gynecology* 46:5 (Nov. 1975):551–56.

Janson, Per Olof, and Inge Jansson. "The Acute Effect of Hysterectomy on Ovarian Blood Flow." *American Journal of Obstetrics and Gynecology* 127:4 (Feb. 1977):349–352.

Madaras, Lynda, and Jane Patterson. *Womancare*. New York: Avon, 1981.

McKeithen, W.S. "Major Gynecologic Survey in Elderly Females 65 Years of Age and Older." *American Journal of Obstetrics and Gynecology* 123:1 (1975):59–65.

McKinlay, John B. "Who Is Really Ignorant—Physician or Patient?" *Journal of Health and Social Behavior*, 16 (1), (March 1975):3–11.

Morris, Louis A., and Jerome A. Halperin. "Effects of Written Drug Information on Patient Knowledge and Compliance: A Literature Review." *American Journal of Public Health* 69:1 (Jan. 1979):47–52.

Paulshock, Bernadine Z. "What Every Woman Should Know About Hysterectomy." *Today's Health* 54:2 (Feb. 1976):23–26.

Ranney, B., and S. Abu-Ghazaleh. "The Future Function and Fortune of Ovarian Tissue Which Is Retained in Vivo During Hysterectomy." *American Journal of Obstetrics and Gynecology* 128:626 (1977).

CHAPTER 6

Page
No.

95.   *graduate school reading level.* T.M. Grundner. "On the Readability of Surgical Consent Forms." *New England Journal of Medicine* 302:16 (April 17, 1980).

109.   *lift yourself to a sitting position.* Dee Dee Jameson, and Roberta Schwalb. *Every Woman's Guide to Hysterectomy: Taking Charge of Your Own Body.* Englewood Cliffs, NJ: Spectrum Books, 1978 (paper).

110.   *In one large study.* D.H. Richards. "A Post-Hysterectomy Syndrome." *The Lancet.* 2(7887) (Oct. 1974):983–985.

ADDITIONAL REFERENCES FOR CHAPTER 6 TAKING IT OUT

Annas, George L. *The Rights of Hospital Patients: An ACLU Handbook.* New York: Avon, 1975.

Burchell, R. Clay. "Counseling in Gynecologic Practice: An Overview." *Clinical Obstetrics and Gynecology.* 21:1 (March 1978):165.

Butts, Priscilla. "Meeting the Special Needs of your Hysterectomy Patient." *Nursing* 79 (Nov.):40–47.

"Governor Brown Signs AB 1752 into Law." (Concerns protection of human subjects in Medical Experimentation). Institute for the Study of Medical Ethics, *ISME Newsletter* (July 1978).

Jeffcoate, T.N.A. "Posterior Colpoperineorrharhy." *American Journal of Obstetrics and Gynecology* 77:3 (March 1959):490–502.

Jequier, Anne M. "Urinary Symptoms and Total Hysterectomy." *British Journal of Urology* 48 (1976):437–441.

Keaveny, Mary Ellen, et al. "Hysterectomy: Helping Patients Adjust." *Nursing* 3:2 (Feb. 1973):8–12.

Laros, Russell K., Jr., and Bruce A Work, Jr. "Female Sterilization III. Vaginal Hysterectomy." *American Journal of Obstetrics and Gynecology* 122:6 (July 1975):693–697.

Lohrenz, F.N., et al. "Evaluation of Post Hysterectomy Patients by Outcome Techniques." *Wisconsin Medical Journal* 74:1 (Jan. 1975):S–11.

Sime, A. Marilyn. "Relationship of Preoperative Fear, Type of Coping, and Information Received About Surgery to Recovery from Surgery." *Journal of Personality and Social Psychology.* 34:4 (1976):716–724.

Steele, S.J., and M.F. Goodwin. "A Pamphlet to Answer the Patient's Questions Before Hysterectomy." *The Lancet* 7933:2 (Sept. 13, 1975): 492–493.

Vernon, Audree. "Explaining Hysterectomy." *Nursing* (Sept. 1973): 36–38.

CHAPTER 7

Page
No.

113. *women who are neither.*

> Doris Menzer et al. "Patterns of Emotional Recovery from Hysterectomy." *Psychosomatic Medicine* 19:5 (1957):379–388.
> Nancy C. A. Roeske. "Quality of Life and Factors Affecting the Response to Hysterectomy." *The Journal of Family Practice* 7:3 (1978):483–488.

114. *Be aware that nurses and doctors.* A good example of this training is Celeste R. Nagel Phillips. "The Hysterectomy Patient in the Obstetrics Service: A Presurgery Class Helps Meet Her Needs." *Journal of Obstetrical and Gynecological Nursing* 6:1 (Jan–Feb. 1977):45–49.

117. *taught to be aware of these anxieties in their patients.*

> R. Clay Burchell. "Counseling in Gynecologic Practice: An Overview." *Clinical Obstetrics and Gynecology* 21:1 (March 1978):165.

Priscilla Butts. "Meeting the Special Needs of Your Hysterectomy Patient." *Nursing* 79 (Nov. 1979):40–47.

Joan Cornish. "Psychodynamics of the Hysterectomy Experience." In McNall and Galeener, eds. *Current Practice in Obstetrics and Gynecological Nursing.* St. Louis: Mosby, 1976.

Bonnie Cosper et al. "Characteristics of Post Hospitalization Recovery Following Hysterectomy." *Journal of Obstetrical and Gynecological Nursing* 7:3 (May–June 1978).

Don Sloan. "The Emotional and Psychosocial Aspect of Hysterectomy." *American Journal of Obstetrics and Gynecology* 131:6 (July 15, 1978).

Marcia L. Storch et al. "Preparation and Education for the Patient Undergoing Hysterectomy." *Quality Review Bulletin* (March 1977):25.

Marcia Walker. "Total Hysterectomy." *Nursing Times* 73:50 (Dec. 15, 1977):1952–1954.

Barry G. Wren. "Counseling the Hysterectomy Patient." *Medical Journal of Australia* (1978):87–89.

117. *parts of her body.* Nancy A. Roeske. "The Emotional Response to Hysterectomy." *Psychiatric Opinion* (Feb. 1978):11–20.

118. *odd not to have them.* Drellich and Bieber; Nancy Roeske.

120. *not being able to have more.* Beverley Raphael; Doris Menzer et al.

120. RESOLVE. RESOLVE Inc. can be reached at P.O. Box 474, Belmont, MA 02718.

120. *"dirty deal."* Drellich and Bieber.

122. *refuse to have intercourse with them.* See especially George F. Melody.

ADDITIONAL REFERENCES FOR CHAPTER 7 FEELINGS, FEARS, AND GRIEF

Barker, Montague G. "Psychiatric Illness After Hysterectomy." *British Medical Journal* 2 (April 1968):91–95.

Baron, Enid, and Niles Newton. "Psychological Effects of Hysterectomy: Review of Empirical Research." Second National Meeting, Special Section of Psychosomatic Obstetrics and Gynecology of the American College of Obstetrics and Gynecology, Northwestern University (Jan. 1974).

Bragg, Robert L. "Risk of Admission to Mental Hospital Following Hysterectomy or Cholescystectomy." *American Journal of Public Health* 55:9 (Sept. 1965):1403–10.

Castelnuovo-Tedesco, Pietro, and Boyd Krout. "Psychosomatic Aspects of Chronic Pelvic Pain." *Psychiatry in Medicine* 1:2 (April 1970): 109–127.

Chynoweth, R. "Psychological Complications of Hysterectomy." *Australian and New Zealand Journal of Psychiatry* 7:102 (June 1973):102–104.

Coope, Jean. "The Post-Hysterectomy Syndrome." *The Lancet* 2:7889 (Nov. 1974):1142.

Cornish, Joan. "Psychodynamics of the Hysterectomy Experience." In McNall and Galeener, eds. *Current Practice in Obstetrical and Gynecological Nursing.* St. Louis: Mosby, 1976.

Cosper, Bonnie, et al. "Characteristics of Posthospitalization Recovery Following Hysterectomy." *Journal of Obstetrical and Gynecological Nursing* 7:3 (May–June 1978).

Dodds, D.T., et al. "The Physical and Emotional Results of Hysterectomy." *South African Medical Journal* 35:3 (Jan. 21, 1961):53–54.

Douglas, Gordon W. "Emotional Problems Associated with Hysterectomy." *Journal of the American Osteopathic Assn.* 70:12 (Aug. 1971): 1345/119–1346/120.

Drellich, Marvin G., and Irving Bieber. "The Psychologic Importance of the Uterus and Its Functions." *Journal of Nervous and Mental Diseases* 126:1 (Jan. 1958):322–336.

Grover, John W. "A Gynecologist's View." *Psychiatric Opinion* (Feb. 1978):21.

Hampton, Peter, and William G. Tarnasky. "Hysterectomy and Tubal Ligation: A Comparison of the Psychological Aftermath." *American Journal of Obstetrics and Gynecology* 119:7 (Aug. 1, 1974):949–52.

Hunter, David J.S. "Effects of Hysterectomy." *The Lancet* 2:7891 (Nov. 1974):1265–66.

Jacobs, Warren M., et al. "The Effect of Hysterectomy on Young Women." *Surgery, Gynecology and Obstetrics* 104:3 (March 1957): 307–309.

Lindemann, Erich. "Observations on Psychiatric Sequelae to Surgical Operations in Women." *American Journal of Psychiatry* 98:1 (1941): 132–139.

Meikle, Stewart, et al. "An Investigation into the Psychological Effects of Hysterectomy." *The Journal of Nervous and Mental Disease* 164:1 (1977):36.

Melody, George F. "Depressive Reactions Following Hysterectomy." *American Journal of Obstetrics and Gynecology* 83:3 (Feb. 1, 1962): 410–413.

Menzer, Doris, et al. "Patterns of Emotional Recovery from Hysterectomy." *Psychosomatic Medicine* 19:5 (1957):379–388.

Mills, Wilfrid G. "Depression After Hysterectomy." *The Lancet* 2:7830 (Sept. 22, 1973):672–673.

Moore, James T., and Dennis H. Tolley. "Depression Following Hysterectomy." *Psychosomatics* 17:2 (1976):86–89.

Newton, Niles, and Enid Baron. "Reactions to Hysterectomy: Fact or Fiction?" *Primary Care* 3:4 (Dec. 1976):781–801.

Newton, Niles. "Psychological Impact of Female Surgery." Speech given at "Women in Conflict" symposium, Chicago Lying-In Hospital, Chicago (Jan. 27, 1976).

Notman, Malkah T., in Bunker et al. "Elective Hysterectomy: Pro and Con." *New England Journal of Medicine* 295:5 (July 29, 1976):266–67.

Osofsky, Howard J., and Robert Seidenberg. "Is Female Menopausal Depression Inevitable?" *Obstetrics and Gynecology* 36:4 (1970):611–615.

Patterson, Ralph M., and James B. Craig. "Misconceptions Concerning the Psychological Effects of Hysterectomy." *American Journal of Obstetrics and Gynecology* 85:1 (Jan. 1, 1963):104.

Phillips, Celeste R. Nagel. "The Hysterectomy Patient in the Obstetrics Service: A Presurgery Class Helps Meet Her Needs." *Journal of Obstetrical and Gynecological Nursing* 6:1 (Jan.–Feb. 1977): 45–49.

Polivy, Janet. "Psychological Reactions to Hysterectomy: A Critical Review." *American Journal of Obstetrics and Gynecology* 118:3 (Feb. 1974):417–426.

Raphael, Beverley. "The Crisis of Hysterectomy." *Australian–New Zealand Journal of Psychiatry* 6:106 (1972).

Richards, D.H. "Depression After Hysterectomy." *The Lancet* 2:7826 (Aug. 25, 1973):430–32.

Richards, D.H. "Effects of Hysterectomy." *The Lancet* 2:7894 (Dec. 1974):1450.

Roeske, Nancy A. "The Emotional Response to Hysterectomy." *Psychiatric Opinion* (Feb. 1978):11–20.

Roeske, Nancy C.A. "Quality of Life and Factors Affecting the Response to Hysterectomy." *The Journal of Family Practice* 7:3 (1978):483–488.

Sloan, Don. "The Emotional and Psychosocial Aspect of Hysterectomy." *American Journal of Obstetrics and Gynecology* 131:6 (July 15, 1978).

Steiner, M., and D.R. Aleksandrowicz. "Psychiatric Sequelae to Gynecological Operations." *The Israel Annals of Psychiatry and Related Disciplines* 8:2 (July 1970):186–193.

Storch, Marcia L., and Maryanne Shanahan. "Preparation and Education for the Patient Undergoing Hysterectomy." Case Report, *Quality Review Bulletin* (March 1977):25.

Walker, Marcia. "Total Hysterectomy." *Nursing Times* 73:50 (Dec. 15, 1977):152–154.

Williams, Margaret Aasterud. "Easier Convalescence." *American Journal of Nursing* 76:3 (March 1976):438–440.

Wren, Barry. "Counseling the Hysterectomy Patient." *Medical Journal of Australia* 1 (1978):87–89.

Zervos, S.K., and Papaloucas, A.C. "Psychosomatic Disturbances Following Hysterectomy Performed at a Premenopausal Age." *International Surgery* 57:10 (Oct. 1972):802–804.

CHAPTER 8

Much of this chapter is based on my article "Sexuality After Hysterectomy and Castration," *Women and Health* 3:1 (Jan.–Feb. 1978).

Page No.

131. *"Sexual gratification is in no way . . ."* Nancy Nugent. *Hysterectomy: A Complete Up-to-date Guide to Everything About It and Why It May Be Needed.* New York: Doubleday, 1976, p. 87.

131. *"The majority of women . . ."* Audree Vernon. "Explaining Hysterectomy." *Nursing 73* (Sept. 1973):37.

132. "*A woman . . .*" William H. Masters and Virginia E. Johnson. "What Young Women Should Know About Hysterectomies." *Redbook* magazine 146:3 (Jan. 1976):50.

132. "*Sex should not feel . . .*" Reimer. *Patient Information Library* (1979).

132. "*Apart from mental and emotional variables . . .*" Lucienne Lanson. *From Woman to Woman* (1978):179.

132. "*For women whose uteruses . . .*" Boston Women's Health Book Collective. *Our Bodies, Ourselves.* 2nd ed. New York: Simon and Schuster, 1976:149.

132. "*There is no relationship . . .*" Dee Dee Jameson and Roberta Schwalb. *Hysterectomy: Taking Charge of Your Body.* Englewood Cliffs, NJ: Spectrum, 1978, p. 119.

132. *Recent research.* Leon Zussman et al. "Sexual Response After Hysterectomy—Oophorectomy: Recent Studies and Reconsideration of Psychogenesis," *American Journal of Obstetrics and Gynecology.* (In press) Reprint requests to Robert Sunley, Family Service Association of Nassau County, 129 Jackson Street, Hempstead, NY 11550.

133. *The stages of female sexual arousal.*

> William H. Masters and Virginia E. Johnson. *Human Sexual Response.* Boston: Little, Brown, 1966.
> Masters and Johnson's work is summarized in R. and E. Brecher. *An Analysis of Human Sexual Response.* Boston: Little, Brown, 1976.
> An additional resource is: I. Singer. *The Goals of Human Sexuality.* New York: Norton, 1973.

138. *two kinds of orgasms.* My great appreciation to Edith Bjornson for this documentation. (Personal communication)

139. *point out the fact that many women.* Cited by Edith Bjornson (personal communication, June 1, 1981)

139. *These orgasms are triggered by.* Zussman et al. Citing Masters, personal communication, L. Clark. "Is There a Difference Be-

tween a Clitoral and a Vaginal Orgasm?" *Journal of Sex Research* 6 (1970):27–30, and Singer.

139. *There may be a relationship.* Zussman et al.

139. *A young man.* Interview by Donelle Dadigan, student at UCLA in CED course "Hysterectomy: An Interdisciplinary Perspective" (Fall 1977).

139. *Eddy's wife.* Interview by Paul Catterton, UCLA (1977).

140. *Does removal.* Lanson, p. 179.

141. *despite Lanson's assertion.* Lanson.

142. *the rate of complication.*

See Donahue, in Bunker, ed. "Elective Hysterectomy: Pro and Con." *New England Journal of Medicine* 295:5 (1976):264.
Lester R. Hubbard. "Sexual Sterilization by Elective Hysterectomy." *American Journal of Obstetrics and Gynecology* 112:8 (1972).
Cedric W. Porter, Jr. and Jaroslav F. Hulka. "Female Sterilization in Current Clinical Practice," *Family Planning Perspective.* 6:1:30–38.
Carl J. Levenson. "Hysterectomy Complications." *Clinical Obstetrics and Gynecology* 15 (Sept. 1972):802–826.

142. *Other documented complications.* Attributed to Nora Coffey by Edith Bjornson (personal communication).

142. *Masters and Johnson.* William H. Masters and Virginia E. Johnson. *Human Sexual Inadequacy.* Boston: Little, Brown, 1970, p. 187.

146. *source of androgen.*

J. Money. "Components of Eroticism in Man: I. The Hormones in Relation to Sexual Morphology and Sexual Desires." *Journal of Nervous and Mental Diseases* 132 (1961):239–248.
U.J. Salmon and S.H. Geist. "Effects of Androgens upon Libido in Women." *Journal of Clinical Endocrinology* 3:235 (1943). Cited in Zussman.

146. *Estrogen replacement does not affect.* W.H. Utian. "Effect of Hysterectomy, Oophorectomy, and Estrogen Therapy on Libido." *International Journal of Gynecology and Obstetrics* 13:97 (1975).

146. *also in the ovaries.*

> R.H. Asch and Greenblatt, R. "Steroidogenesis in the Post-Menopausal Ovary." *Clinical Obstetrics and Gynecology* 4:1 (1977):85. Cited in Zussman.
>
> Studd and Thom. "Ovarian Failure and Aging." *Clinics in Endocrinology and Metabolism* 10:1 W.B. Saunders (March 1981), from Edith Bjornson (personal communication).

146. *"masculinizing" changes.* Robert B. Greenblatt and Jean C. Emperaire. "Changing Concepts in the Medical Management of the Menopause." *Medical Times* 98:6 (June 1970):153–164.

146. *androgen pellets.* Thom and Studd. "Hormone Implantation." *British Medical Journal* (March 22, 1980), from Edith Bjornson (personal communication).

146. *the prescription for home-brew.* See Chapter 9.

147. *castration of female animals.*

> John C. Money. "Psychosexual differentiation." in Money, ed. *Sex Research: New Developments.* New York: Holt, Rinehart and Winston, 1965, pp. 16–17.
>
> Richard P. Michael and D. Zumpe. "Aggression and Gonadal Hormones in Captive Rhesus Monkeys." *Animal Behavior* 18 (1980):1–10.

147. *human pheromones.*

> Robert Schneider. "The Sense of Smell and Human Sexuality," *Medical Aspects of Human Sexuality* (May 1971):157–168.
>
> "More Evidence for Human Sex Pheromones." *Science News* 109 (Jan. 3, 1976):6.
>
> Richard L. Doty et al. "Changes in the Intensity and Pleasantness of Human Vaginal Odors During the Menstrual Cycle." *Science* 190 (Dec. 26, 1975):1316–1318.

153. *Few studies.* A good summary of these studies is Niles Newton and Enid Baron. "Reactions to Hysterectomy: Fact or Fiction." *Primary Care* 3:4 (Dec. 1976):781–801.

154. Table source: Zussman.
Studies cited are:

> D.R. Richards, "A Post-Hysterectomy Syndrome." *The Lancet* 2 (1974):982.
>
> G.A. Craig and P. Jackson. "Sexual Life After Vaginal Hysterectomy." *British Medical Journal* 1 (1975):97.
>
> W.H. Utian. "Effect of Hysterectomy, Oophorectomy and Estrogen Therapy on Libido." *International Journal of Gynaecology and Obstetrics* 13 (1975):97.
>
> L. Dennerstein et al. "Sexual Responses Following Hysterectomy and Oophorectomy." *Obstetrics and Gynaecology* 49 (1977):92.
>
> S. Chakravarti et al. "Endocrine Changes and Symptomatology After Oophorectomy in Premenopausal Women." *British Journal of Obstetrics and Gynaecology* 84 (1977):767.

153. *Since the operation.* Peter T. Hampton and William G. Tarnasky. "Hysterectomy and Tubal Ligation: A Comparison of the Psychological Aftermath," *American Journal of Obstetrics and Gynecology* 119:7 (Aug. 1, 1974):949–952.

153. *Not all studies of psychological.* Polivy's review is a disappointing example. Janet Polivy. "Psychological Reactions to Hysterectomy: A Critical Review." *American Journal of Obstetrics and Gynecology* 118:3 (Feb. 1, 1974):417–426.

155. *women who were unmarried.* John C. Burch et al. "The Effects of Long-Term Estrogen on Hysterectomized Women." *American Journal of Obstetrics and Gynecology* 118:6 (March 15, 1974): 778–782.

155. *they are retrospective.* Zussman.

155. *"sexual gratification . . ."* Nugent, p. 87.

155. *Masters and Johnson describe.* Masters and Johnson. *Human Sexual Inadequacy,* p. 187.

155. *"Eight . . . continued to state . . ."* Diana Scully and Pauline Bart. "A Funny Thing Happened on the Way to the Orifice: Women in Gynecology Textbooks." *American Journal of Sociology* 78:4 (1973):1048.

156. *Gail Whitman.* Gail F. Whitman. "Sexual Sequelae of Cervical Cancer and Its Therapy: A Preliminary Research Report." Presented at meetings of the International Society of Psychosomatic Obstetrics and Gynaecology (April 9, 1976).

156. *Shere Hite's survey.* Shere Hite. *The Hite Report.* New York: Macmillan, 1976.

157. *husband's reaction.* Masters and Johnson, 1967, p. 51.

157. *"support, encourage, and counsel . . ."* Paul D. Mozley. "Woman's Capacity for Orgasm after Menopause." *Medical Aspects of Human Sexuality* 9:8 (Aug. 1975):104, 109, 110.

157. *In two major studies*

   Nancy Nugent. *Hysterectomy: A Complete Up-to-Date Guide to Everything About It and Why It May Be Needed.* Garden City, New York: Doubleday, 1976, p. 87.

   Marvin G. Drellich and Irving Bieber. "The Psychologic Importance of the Uterus and Its Functions." *Journal of Nervous and Mental Diseases* 126:1 (Jan. 1958):322–336.

157. *Paulshock.* Paulshock, p. 26 (her ellipses).

158. *"So, do not listen . . ."* Paulshock, p. 23.

158. *"It is sometimes hard . . ."* Masters. *Redbook* magazine.

159. *"Even conversations . . ."* Nugent, p. 155.

159. *"Erroneous notions . . ."* A.G. Amais. "Sexual Life After Gynaecological Operations—I." *British Medical Journal* 5971 (June 14, 1975):609. See also the exchange following the article: Letters, *British Medical Journal* (Aug. 9, 1975):368.

159. *An article in the January 1979.* Louis A. Morris and Jerome A. Halperin. "Effects of Written Drug Information on Patient Knowledge and Compliance: A Literature Review." *American Journal of Public Health* 69:1 (Jan. 1979):47–52.

160. *Two articles . . . document improved detection.* The articles are in the August 10, 1978 issue of the *New England Journal of Medicine,* and the analysis was presented by Diane Turkin in a letter to the National Women's Health Network.

161. *Recently researchers investigating language.* John B. McKinlay. "Who Is Really Ignorant—Physician or Patient?" *Journal of Health and Social Behavior* 16:1 (March 1975):3–11.

162. *The medical profession . . .* K. Jean Lennane and R. John Lennane. "Alleged Psychogenic Disorders in Women: A Possible Manifestation of Sexual Prejudice." *The New England Journal of Medicine* 288 (Feb. 1, 1973):288.

162. *Effects of hysterectomy on sexuality.* Zussman et al. present this powerfully.

163. *"If a woman complains . . ."* Masters and Johnson, *Human Sexual Inadequacy,* p. 288.

163. *"However, if a woman discovers . . ."* William Masters. *Redbook* magazine, p. 50.

165. *"The generally accepted . . ."* Martin L. Madorsky. "Sexual function After Orchietomy." *Medical Aspects of Human Sexuality* (Dec. 1975):59.

165. *Another example is the contrast.* "Treating Menopausal Women—and Climacteric Men." *Medical World News* 15 (June 1974): 37–44.

166. *re-evaluation co-counseling.* Information about groups in your area can be obtained by writing 719 Second Avenue North, Seattle, WA 98109.

167. *For Yourself: The Fulfillment of Female Sexuality* by Lonnie Garfield Barbach. New York: Doubleday, 1975; New York: Signet, 1976 (paper).

CHAPTER 9

**Page
No.**

171. *Dangers of Estrogen.* The National Institute of Health Consensus Development Conference on Estrogen Use and Post-Menopausal Women (September 13 and 14, 1979) summarized the most up-to-date information on risks and benefits of estrogen. You can write for a copy from the Office for Medical Applications of Research, National Institute of Health, Building 1, Room 216, Bethesda, MD 20205.

171. *Endometrial cancer occurs more often.*

> Carolos M.F. Antunes et al. "Endometrial Cancer and Estrogen Use." *The New England Journal of Medicine* 300:1 (Jan. 4, 1979):9–13.
>
> Jack Gordon et al. "Estrogen and Endometrial Carcinoma." *The New England Journal of Medicine* (Sept. 15, 1977).
>
> L.A. Gray et al. "Estrogens and Endometrial Carcinoma." *Obstetrics and Gynecology* 49 (1977):385–9.
>
> S.B. Gusberg. "The Changing Nature of Endometrial Cancer." *New England Journal of Medicine* 302:13 (March 27, 1980).
>
> Barbara Hulka. "Effects of Exogenous Estrogen on Postmenopausal Women: The Epidemiologic Evidence." *Obstetrical and Gynecological Survey* 35:6 (1980):389–399.
>
> H. Jick et al. "Replacement Estrogens and Endometrial Cancer." *New England Journal of Medicine* 300 (1979):218–22.
>
> Thomas W. McDonald. *American Journal of Obstetrics and Gynecology,* 127:6 (March 15, 1977):572–580.
>
> National Institute of Health. "Estrogen Use and Post Menopausal Women: Consensus Conference Summary." 2:8 (1980).
>
> Isaac Schiff, and Kenneth J. Ryan. "Benefits of Estrogen Replacement." *Obstetrical and Gynecological Survey* 35:6 (1980):400–410.
>
> Donald C. Smith et al. "Association of Exogenous Estrogen

and Endometrial Carcinoma." *New England Journal of Medicine,* 293:23 (Dec. 4, 1975):1164–1199.

Milton C. Weinstein. "Estrogen Use and Postmenopausal Women: Costs, Risks and Benefits." *New England Journal of Medicine* 303:6 (Aug. 7, 1980):308–316.

Noel S. Weiss. "Risks and Benefits of Estrogen Use." *The New England Journal of Medicine* 293:23 (Dec. 1975).

Noel S. Weiss. "Increasing Incidence of Endometrial Cancer in the U.S." *New England Journal of Medicine* 294:23 (June 3, 1976):1259–67.

173. *progestin's safety.* Stanley G. Korenman. *New England Journal of Medicine* (letters section) 302:5 (Jan. 31, 1980):297.

173. *association between estrogen and breast cancer.*

Robert Hoover et al. "Menopausal Estrogens and Breast Cancer." *The New England Journal of Medicine* 295:8 (Aug. 19, 1976):401–405.

Hulka reviews this research.

Sidney M. Wolfe. "Evidence of Breast Cancer from DES and Current Prescribing of DES and Other Estrogens." Paper presented before FDA OB-GYN Advisory Committee (Jan. 30, 1978).

173. *gallbladder disease.*

Boston Collaborative Drug Surveillance Program, Boston University Medical Center. *New England Journal of Medicine* 296 (1977):716–21.

National Institute of Health. "Estrogen Use . . ."

174. *women request.*

Robert A. Wilson. *Feminine Forever.* New York: Evans, 1966.

Lila Nachtigall with Joan Heilman. *The Lila Nachtigall Report.* New York: Putnam, 1977.

174. *Only with books like.*

Rosetta Reitz. *Menopause: A Positive Approach.* Radnor, Pa.: Clilton Books, 1977; New York: Penguin, 1979 (paper).

Barbara and Gideon Seaman. *Women and the Crisis in Sex Hormones.* New York: Rawson, 1977; New York: Bantam, 1978.

174. *ads for ERT products.* Seaman, Chapter 22 (hardcover p. 281).

175. *letter from Hill and Knowlton.* Sharon Lieberman. "New Discovery: Public Relations Cures Cancer." *Majority Report* (Feb. 1977).

176. *results to consumers and legislators.*

> Anita Johnson. "The Risks of Sex Hormones as Drugs." *Women and Health* (July–Aug. 1977):8–11.
> "Estrogen Therapy: Dangerous Road to Shangri-La." *Consumer Reports* 41:11 (Nov. 1976):642.

177. *The ovaries are not the only source.*

> J.M. Grodin et al. "Source of Estrogen Production in Post Menopausal Women." *Journal of Clinical Endocrinology and Metabolism,* 36:2 (1973):207.

In 1973 J. M. Grodin, P. K. Siiteri, and P. C. McDonald, working together at the University of Texas in Dallas, showed that among a group of postmenopausal women they studied, they found higher levels of estrogen than they had expected and that the estrogen was not all coming directly from the ovaries. They surmised that as the chemical changes that will ultimately result in estrogen production by the ovary and adrenal glands take place, some of the partially processed hormones in the form of androstenedione leaks out of the ovary and adrenal cells into the bloodstream and the final chemical step to estrogen production takes place in the fat cells. Other researchers have established that this also takes place in the muscle cells, liver cells, and some brain cells.

Page
No.

179. *traditional medical understanding.* The Feminist Women's Health Centers, a nationwide network of women's clinics, have produced a mammoth book called *Women's Health in Women's Hands.* The chapter called "A New View of a Woman's Body" reinterprets much of what we know about hormones. The book is in press and references are to a draft.

179. *fatty tissue under the skin.* Grodin cited in *Women's Health in Women's Hands*, p. 172.

179. *Heavier women.* Barbara Seaman, personal communication (Aug. 27, 1980).

179. *Hormones are produced in the adrenals.* R.W. Kistner. *Gynecology: Principles and Practice.* 2nd ed. Chicago: Yearbook Medical Publishers, 1971, Chapter 13.

180. *Dr. Kurt W. Donsbach.* Kurt W. Donsbach and Alan H. Nittler, *Hysterectomy.* International Institute of Natural Health Sciences, P.O. Box 5550, Huntington Beach, Cal. 92646 (1978).

181. *weakens the adrenals. Women's Health in Women's Hands.* Chapter titled "A New View of a Woman's Body," p. 194, citing:

Paavo Airola. *Hypoglycemia—A Better Approach,* Phoenix: Health Plus, 1978.
K.J. Catt. *An ABC of Endocrinology.* Boston: Little, Brown, 1971.
Jeremy Brecher. "Sex, Stress, and Health." *International Journal of Health Services.* 7:1 (1977).

182. *The bad effects of coffee.* Rosetta Reitz is very adamant on this. Rosetta Reitz. *Menopause: A Positive Approach.*

184. *If you perceive hot flashes.* I recommend highly two books that have a great deal of information on specific alternatives to estrogen:

Rosetta Reitz. *Menopause: A Positive Approach.* New York: Penguin 1977 (paper).
Seaman and Seaman, *Women and the Crisis in Sex Hormones.*

184. *Many people probably take.* Barbara Seaman, personal communication (Aug. 27, 1980).

185. *Ginseng is a root.* Barbara and Gideon Seaman include a chapter with a great deal of information on ginseng in *Women and the Crisis in Sex Hormones.*

186. *"senile vaginal atrophy."* The Feminist Women's Health Center attribute the vaginal changes to poor health.

If physicians find an atrophic condition in an older woman's vagina, they attribute it to ovarian atrophy which they incorrectly think occurs as a result of menopause. It seems more logical to attribute it to ill health since the young women who undergo surgical castration while still menstruating do not necessarily get atrophy of the vagina. (*A New View*, p. 203, draft)

Page
No.

188.   *Two articles claim evidence from animal studies.* Norma Besch et al. "The Effect of Marihuana (Delta-9-Tetrahydrocannabinol) on the Secretions of Luteinizing Hormone in the Ovariectomized Rhesus Monkey." *American Journal of Obstetrics and Gynecology* 128:6 (July 15, 1977):635–642; and Jolane Solomon et al. "Uterotropic Effect of Delta-9-Tetrahydrocannabinol in Ovariectomized Rats." *Science* 192:4239 (May 7, 1976):559–561.

188.   *Functioning well sexually.* Lonnie Garfield Barbach. *For Yourself: the Fulfillment of Female Sexuality.* New York: Signet, 1975. This book has excellent suggestions for relearning how to pleasure ourselves.

189.   *approximately 25 percent of all white women.* Robert P. Heaney. Menopausal Effects on Calcium Homeostasis and Skeletal Metabolism in *Menopause and Aging.* Kenneth Ryan, ed. DHEW Pub. No. (NIH) 73–319 (1971).

189.   *"disease of theories."* Wulf H. Utian. *Menopause in Modern Perspective: A Guide to Clinical Practice.* Appleton-Century-Crofts 1980: p. 73.

189.   *retard bone loss.* Kenneth J. Ryan et al. *Annals of Internal Medicine* 91:921 (1979).

189.   *can accelerate.* R. Lindsay et al. "Bone Response to Termination of Oestrogen Treatment." *The Lancet* 1:1325 (June 24, 1978).

190.   *Nachtigall.* Lila Nachtigall and Joan Heilman. *The Lila Nachtigall Report.* New York: Putnam, 1977.

190. *delay bone loss.* Robert R. Recker, et al. "Effect of Estrogens and Calcium Carbonate on Bone Loss in Postmenopausal Women." *Annals of Internal Medicine* 87:6 (Dec. 1977):649–655.

190. *large doses.* The Medical Letter, Drugs for Postmenopausal Osteoporosis, 22:2 (issue 558) (May 30, 1980):46.

190. *Late evening dose.* Utian, p. 81.

190. *exercise can help.* The Medical Letter, p. 46. J.F. Aloia et al."Prevention of Involutional Bone Loss by Exercise." *Annals of Internal Medicine* 89:356 (1978).

191. *The body's real estrogen.* Women's Health in Women's Hands, draft, "A New View of a Woman's Body," p. 209.

192. *Lila Nachtigall.* The quote is from *Family Circle* magazine, in 1977, and Nachtigall says, "I believe estrogen does *not* cause cancer if it is used properly . . ." Later she says, "I believe that properly administered estrogen replacement . . . does not cause endometrial cancer. In fact, it may even help to prevent it." Lila Nachtigall and Joan Heilman. "Now the Good News About Estrogen." *Family Circle* (Nov. 15, 1977):124.

192. *If you smoke cigarettes.* H.W. Daniell. "Osteoporosis of the Slender Smoker." *Archives of Internal Medicine* 136:298 (1976).

194. *"I have found lots of women . . ."* Rosetta Reitz, personal communication (Aug. 27, 1980).

ADDITIONAL REFERENCES FOR CHAPTER 9
HOME-BREW ESTROGEN

Abe, Tetsuro, et al. "Correlation Between Climacteric Symptoms and Serum Levels of Estradiol, Progesterone, Follicle-Stimulating Hormone, and Luteinizing Hormone." *American Journal of Obstetrics and Gynecology* 129:65 (Sept. 1, 1977):65–67.

Abraham, Guy E., and George B. Maroulis. "Effects of Exogenous Estrogen on Serum Pregnenolone, Cortisol, and Androgens on Postmenopausal Women." *Obstetrics and Gynecology* 45:3 (March 1975): 271–74.

Aitken, J.M., et al. "The Relationship Between Menopausal Vasomotor Symptoms and Gonadotrophin Excretion in Urine After Oophorectomy." *The Journal of Obstetrics and Gynaecology of the British Commonwealth.* 81 (Feb. 1974):150–154.

Aitken, J.M., et al. "Long-Term Oestrogens for the Prevention of Post-Menopausal Osteoporosis." *Postgraduate Medical Journal* 52 (Suppl. 6) (1976):18–25.

Block, Marilyn R., et al. "Uncharted Territory: Issues and Concerns of Women over 40." *Center on Aging.* University of Maryland (1978).

Blanc, Jean-Jacques, et al. "Menopause and Myocardial Infarction." *American Journal of Obstetrics and Gynecology* 127:4 (Feb. 15, 1977):353–355.

Burch, John C., et al. "The Effects of Long-Term Estrogen on Hysterectomized Women." *American Journal of Obstetrics and Gynecology* 118:6 (March 15, 1974):778–782.

Byrd, Benjamin F., et al. "Significance of Postoperative Estrogen Therapy on the Occurrence and Clinical Course of Cancer." *Annals of Surgery* 177:5 (May 1973):626–631.

Cali, Robert W. "Management of the Climacteric and Postmenopausal Women." *Medical Clinics of North America* 56:3 (May 1972):789–800.

Cooper, Wendy. *No Change.* London: Arrow Books, 1976.

Corea, Gena. Letter to *Family Circle* magazine about Lila Nachtigall Report, Network News, National Women's Health Network.

Cowan, Belita. "Menopause—Fact Sheet." *Women's Health Care.*

Dietz, Jean. "A New Use for Estrogen to Help Older Women." *Boston Globe* (Oct. 1, 1978).

Dixon, Marden G. "Female Hormones: Hazardous Panacea." *Trial* magazine (Oct. 1976).

Donald R.A., et al. "Assessment of Ovarian Function in Perimenopausal Women after Stopping Oral Contraceptives." *British Journal of Obstetrics and Gynaecology* 85 (Jan. 1978):70–73.

———. "Effects of Calcium Infusions in Patients with Postmenopausal Osteoporosis." *Metabolism* 24:7 (July 1975):849–54.

———. "Estrogens and Endometrial Cancer." *FDA Drug Bulletin* (Feb./ March 1976).

———. "Estrogens OK for Osteoporosis prevention . . . but 'Imprudent' for DES Women." *Medical World News* (Oct. 30, 1978).

———. "Estrogen Replacement Therapy Is Debated at AMA Meeting." *OB-GYN News* (Aug. 1, 1977).

Flint, Marcha P. "Transcultural Influences in Peri-Menopausal." In Haspels, *Psychosomatics, in Peri-Menopause,* p. 41.

———. "Estrogen Therapy: The Dangerous Road to Shangri-La." *Consumer Reports* (Nov. 1976): 642–645.

Galton, Lawrence. "Estrogen for Menopause—Easing Pain—Without Fear." *Parade* (Aug. 27, 1978).

Gordon, Jack, et al. "Estrogen and Endometrial Carcinoma." *New England Journal of Medicine* 297:11 (Sept. 15, 1977):570–71.

Greenblatt, Robert B., and Jean C. Emperaire. "Changing Concepts in the Management of Menopause." *Medical Times* 98:6 (June 1970): 153–164.

Greenblatt, Robert B., et al. "Treating Menopausal Women and Climacteric Men." *Medical World News* (June 28, 1974):32–44.

Grills, Norma J. "Nutritional Needs of Elderly Women." *Clinical Obstetrics and Gynecology* 20:1 (March 1977): 137–143.

Grody, Marvin H., et al. "Estrogen-Androgen Substitution Therapy in the Aged Female." Uterine Bioassay Report, *Obstetrics and Gynecology* 2:1 (July 1953):36–45.

Hodgen, Gary D., et al. "Menopause in Rhesus Monkeys: Model for Study of Disorders in the Human Climacteric." *American Journal of Obstetrics and Gynecology* 127:6 (March 15, 1977):581–584.

Hollo, I., et al. "Osteoporosis and Androgens." *The Lancet* (June 19, 1976).

Haspels, A.A., and H. Musaph, eds. *Psychosomatics in Peri-Menopause.* Baltimore: University Park Press, 1979.

Haspels, A.A., and P.A. Van Keep. "Endocriminology and Management of the Peri-Menopause." In Haspels, *Psychosomatics*, p. 57.

Hoover, Robert, et al. "Menopausal Estrogens and Breast Cancer." *Obstetrics and Gynecologic Survey* 32:1 (Jan. 1977):55–57.

Horwitz, Ralph I., and Alvan R. Feinstein. "Alternative Analytic Methods for Case-Control Studies of Estrogens and Endometrial Cancer." *The New England Journal of Medicine* 299:20 (Nov. 16, 1978): 1089–1094.

Judd, Howard L., et al. "Endocrine Function of the Postmenopausal Ovary: Concentration of Androgens and Estrogens in Ovarian and Peripheral Vein Blood." *Journal of Clinical Endocriminology and Metabolism* 39:6 (Dec. 1974):1020–1023.

Kannel, William B., et al. "Menopause and Risk of Cardiovascular Disease (The Framingham Study)." *Annals of Internal Medicine* 85:4 (1976):447–456.

Kasper, Anne S. "FDA Requires Estrogen Risk Information." *Women's Washington Report* (Oct. 12, 1977).

Kerr, M. Dorothea. "Psychohormonal Treatment During the Menopause." *AFP* 11:2 (Feb. 1975):99–103.

Lake, Alice. "Our Own Years: What Women over 35 Should Know About Themselves." *Woman's Day.* New York: Random House, 1979.

Lamb, Wanda M., et al. "Premenstrual Tension: EEG, Hormonal, and Psychiatric Evaluation." *American Journal of Psychiatry* 109 (May 1953):840–48.

Lichten, Edward M. "Estrogen and Alternative Therapy to the Menopausal Patient." *Primary Care* 5:4 (Dec. 1978):607–614.

Lindsay, R., et al. "Long-Term Prevention of Post-Menopausal Osteoporosis by Estrogen." *The Lancet* (May 15, 1976):1038–1041.

Lindsay, R., et al. "Duration of Estrogen Therapy to Prevent Bone Loss Uncertain." *Modern Medicine* (Dec. 15, 1978–Jan. 15, 1979).

―――. "Menopause" (Fact Sheet). Berkeley Women's Health Collective.

―――. "Menopause" (Pamphlet). San Francisco Women's Health Center (June 1974; rev. April 1975, Jan. 1976).

Moore, Benjamin. "Sequential Menstranol and Norethisterone in the Treatment of the Climacteric Syndrome." *Postgraduate Medical Journal* 52 (Suppl. 6) (1976):39–46.

MacKenzie, Robert D., et al. "The Effect on Blood Coagulation of Ovariectomy and Hysterectomy in Rats Given Ethinyl Estradiol." *American Journal of Obstetrics and Gynecology* (April 15, 1974): 1041–1049.

McKinlay, Sonja, and John B. McKinlay. "Selected Studies of the Menopause" (Annotated Bibliography). *Journal of Biosociological Science* 5 (1973):533–555.

Pfeffer, R.I. "Estrogen Use in Postmenopausal Women." *American Journal of Epidemiology* 105:1 (1977):21–29.

Pratt, Marilynn J. "Progesterone—The Sleeper in Female Health (Paper). Women's Institute and Health Center, Inc., 7151 W. Manchester Ave., Los Angeles, CA 90045.

―――. "Estrogen (the Stepchild of Medicine) Seeks Adoption and Understanding" (Paper). Women's Institute and Health Center, Inc.

Richards, N.A. "The Surgical Menopause Following Hysterectomy: A Study of 332 Cases." *Proceedings of the Royal Society of Medicine* 44:6 (June 1951):496–97.

Rosenberg, Lynn. "Myocardial Infarction and Estrogen Therapy in Post-Menopausal Women." *New England Journal of Medicine* 294:3 (June 3, 1976):1256–1258.

Ross, R. K., et al. "A Case-Control Study of Menopausal Estrogen Therapy and Breast Cancer." *Journal of the American Medical Association* 198:243; 165–9.

Seidlitz, Sarah. "The Menopause—A Selective Bibliography." Berkeley Women's Health Collective (May 1976).

Shoemaker, Stanton, et al. "Estrogen Treatment of Postmenopausal Women." *JAMA* 238:14 (Oct. 13, 1977):1524–30.

Solomon, Joan. "Menopause: A Rite of Passage." *Ms.* magazine

Solomon, Jolane, et al. "Uterotropic Effect of Delta-9-Tetrahydrocannabinol in Ovariectomized Rats." *Science* 192:4239 (May 7, 1976): 559.

Sturdee, D.W., et al. "Hot Flashes and Estrogen Therapy." Letter in *The Lancet* (July 17, 1976).

Tzingoumis, Vassilias A., et al. "Estriol in the Management of the Menopause." *JAMA* 239:16 (April 21, 1978):1638–41.

———. "Using Fluoride to Curb Osteoporosis." *Medical World News* (Jan. 18, 1974).

———. "Using Premarin (Conjugated Estrogens Tablets, U.S.P.) Today." Pamphlet by Ayerst Laboratories, N.Y. (rev. Nov. 1976).

Utian, Wulf H. "Current Status of Menopause and Postmenopausal Estrogen Therapy." *Obstetrical and Gynecological Survey* 32:4 (1977):193–204.

Williams, C.W.L. "Clonidine in Treatment of Menopausal Flushing." *The Lancet* 7816:1 (June 16, 1973):1388.

Winokur, George. "Depression in the Menopause." *American Journal of Psychiatry* 130:1 (Jan. 1973):92–93.

Wolfe, Sidney. Presentation of Public Citizen's Health Research Group to FDA Advisory Committee on the Use of Estrogens During Menopause (Dec. 16, 1975).

Wolfe, Sidney J. Letter to Alexander M. Schmidt, *Public Citizen.* Health Research Group (Jan. 8, 1976).

Zahn, Debbie. "Is Estrogen Worth Cancer Risk?" *Daily Breeze* (Torrance, CA) (April 24, 1978).

SOURCE NOTES- APPENDIX I

ALTERNATIVE HEALING METHODS

Page No.

209. *Among professional healers.* MacTaggart and MacTaggart. *The Health Care Dilemma.* Mosby, 1976.

210. *Overview of self-care.* Donald B. Ardel. *High Level Wellness.* Emmaeus, PA: Rodale Press, 1977.

210. *A good basic resource.* Mark Bricklin. *The Practical Encyclopaedia of Natural Healing.* Emmaeus, PA: Rodale Press, 1976.

210. *Kay Weiss.* Kay Weiss, ed. *Women's Medicine: Alternative Treatments.* Reston Pub. Co., 1982 (in press)

213. *My favorite books on menopause.*

Barbara Seaman and Gideon Seaman, *Women and the Crisis in Sex Hormones.* Rawson, 1977; Bantam, 1978 (paper).
Rosetta Reitz. *Menopause: A Positive Approach.* Radnor, PA: Chilton Books, 1977; Penguin, 1979 (paper).

214. *Encyclopedia-style book of herbs.* William Hulton. *The Rodale Herb Book.* Emmaeus, PA: Rodale Publishing Co.

214. *Information on diet.* Paavo Airola. *Hypoglycemia—A Better Approach.* Phoenix: Health Plus, 1978.

214. *Visualization.* Mike Samuels and Hal Bennett. *The Well Body Book.* New York: Random House/Bookworks, 1973.

215. *Reflexology.*

>   Mildred Carter. *Hand Reflexology.* West Nyack, NY: Parker, 1975.
>   Mildred Carter. *Helping Yourself with Foot Reflexology.*

215. *Touch for Health.* Local contacts can be found by writing the Touch for Health Foundation at 1174 North Lake Ave., Pasadena, CA 91104.

SOURCE NOTES- APPENDIX II

THE PSYCHOLOGICAL RESEARCH ON HYSTERECTOMY

Page
No.
219. *hard question.* Enid Baron, and Niles Newton. Northwestern University, Psychological Effects of Hysterectomy: Review of Empirical Research, Second National Meeting—Special Section of Psychosomatic Obstetrics and Gynecology of the American College of Obstetrics and Gynecology (January 1974).

219. *short questions.*

John C. Burch, et al. "The Effects of Long-Term Estrogen on Hysterectomized Women." *American Journal of Obstetrics and Gynecology* 118:6 (March 15, 1974):778–782.
R. Chynoweth. "Psychological Complications of Hysterectomy." *Australian and New Zealand Journal of Psychiatry* 7:102 (June 1973):102–104.
D.T. Dodds et al. "The Physical and Emotional Results of Hysterectomy." *South African Medical Journal* 35:3 (Jan. 21, 1961):53–54.
Peter Hampton and William G. Tarnasky. "Hysterectomy and Tubal Ligation: A Comparison of the Psychological After-

math." *American Journal of Obstetrics and Gynecology* 119:7 (Aug. 1, 1974):949–952.

Stewart Meikle et al. "An Investigation Into the Psychological Effects of Hysterectomy." *The Journal of Nervous and Mental Diseases* 164:1 (1977):36–41.

Ralph M. Patterson and James B. Craig. "Misconceptions Concerning the Psychological Effects of Hysterectomy." *American Journal of Obstetrics and Gynecology* 85:1 (Jan. 1, 1963):104.

219. *in-depth interviews.*

Marvin G. Drellich and Irving Bieber. "The Psychologic Importance of the Uterus and Its Functions." *Journal of Nervous and Mental Diseases* 126:1 (Jan. 1958):322–336.

Beverley Raphael. "The Crisis of Hysterectomy." *New Zealand Journal of Psychiatry* 6:106 (1972).

220. *follow-up study.* Bruce C. Richards. "Hysterectomy: From Women to Women." *American Journal of Obstetrics and Gynecology* 131:4 (June 15, 1978):446–452.

221. *first study.* D.H. Richards. "Depression After Hysterectomy." *The Lancet* (Oct. 1973):918–919.

222. *second study.*

D.H. Richards. "Effects of Hysterectomy." *The Lancet* 2:7894 (Dec. 1974):1450.

D.H. Richards. "A Post-Hysterectomy Syndrome." *The Lancet* 2:7887 (Oct. 1974):983–985.

224. *Drellich and.* Marvin G. Drellich and Irving Bieber. "The Psychologic Importance of the Uterus and Its Functions," *Journal of Nervous and Mental Diseases* 126:1 (Jan. 1958):322–336.

225. *complete female.* Drellich and Bieber, p. 323.

226. *all the time.* Drellich and Bieber, p. 326.

227. *psychiatric illness.* Montague G. Barker: "Psychiatric Illness After Hysterectomy." *British Medical Journal* 2 (April 1968):91–95.

229. *"Elective hysterectomy."* Enid Baron and Niles Newton. "Reactions to Hysterectomy: Fact or Fiction?" *Primary Care* 3:4 (Dec. 1976):781–801.

The following references have also been helpful in preparing this material:

————. "The Emotional Response to Hysterectomy." *Psychiatric Opinion* (Feb. 1978):11–20.

Bragg, Robert L. "Risk of Admission to Mental Hospital Following Hysterectomy or Cholecystectomy." *American Journal of Public Health* 55:9 (Sept. 1965):1403–1410.

Lindemann, Erich. "Observations on Psychiatric Sequelae to Surgical Operations in Women." *American Journal of Psychiatry* 98:1 (1941): 132–139.

Melody, George F. "Depressive Reactions Following Hysterectomy." *American Journal of Obstetrics and Gynecology* 83:3 (Feb. 1, 1962): 410–413.

Polivy, Janet. "Psychological Reactions to Hysterectomy: A Critical Review." *American Journal of Obstetrics and Gynecology* 118:3 (Feb. 1974):417–426.

Roeske, Nancy C.A. "Quality of Life and Factors Affecting the Response to Hysterectomy." *The Journal of Family Practice* 7:3 (1978):483–488.

INDEX